Transplants: Unwrapping the Second Gift of Life

The inside story of transplants as told by recipients and their families, donor families, and health professionals

Pat Stave Helmberger

Transplants: Unwrapping the Second Gift of Life: The Inside Story of Organ Transplants as Told by Recipients and Their Families, Donor Families, and Health Professionals ©1992 by Pat Stave Helmberger

All rights reserved. Except for brief passages used for review purposes, no part of this publication may be reproduced, stored in a retrieval system, or transmitted, in any form or by any means, electronic photocopying, recording, or otherwise, without the prior written permission of CHRONIMED Publishing.

Library of Congress Cataloging-in-Publication Data

Helmberger, Pat Stave
    Transplants: unwrapping the second gift of life/Pat Stave Helmberger
            p.   cm.
    ISBN 1-56561-004-0 : $9.95
    1. Transplantation of organs, tissues, etc.--Popular works.
    2. Transplantation of organs, tissues, etc.--Patients--Interviews.
I. Title
  RD120.75.H45 1992
  362.1'9795--dc20
                                  92-5635
                                      CIP

Edited by: Donna Hoel
Cover Design: Eric Lecy
Printed in the United States of America

10 9 8 7 6 5 4 3 2 1

Published by
CHRONIMED Publishing
P.O. Box 47945
Minneapolis, MN 55447-9727

Dedication

This book is dedicated to my sisters Ardelle, Marilyn, and Marion, to the people whose stories inspired this book, to all donor families everywhere, and to the thousands who wait for a second chance at life.

Transplants: Unwrapping the Second Gift of Life

Contents

Introduction 9
Prologue: Where the Journey Began 13

1. Ardelle: A Change of Heart 19
2. Bill: Love Takes a Detour 39
3. Ardelle: Homecoming 55
4. Betty and Wesley: Trading Up 59
5. Connie: Facing Fears, Celebrating Joys 79
6. Mary: A Journey of Love 87
7. Cal: Charting a New Course 107
8. Larry: Sailing for Strength 115
9. Ardelle: Trouble on the Road 121
10. Kelly, Crosby, and Mary: Travel Guides 131
11. Robert: Tackling Roadblocks 145
12. Rick: A Donor Family's Tragedy 151
13. Bob: Unacknowledged Grief 159
14. Mary and Tom: Keepers of the Bridge 171
15. Juliette: Making the Journey Count 179
16. Arthur: Ethics in the New Frontier 187
17. Ardelle: The Journey Comes Full Circle 193

Epilogue: Saying Farewell 203

Transplants: Unwrapping the Second Gift of Life

ACKNOWLEDGEMENTS

The seed of this book grew out of my sister Ardelle's brave decision to accept the heart of a stranger. To her goes my deep gratitude for giving me and other family members the joy of her extended life with us. And to my sisters, Marilyn and Marion, go my thanks for their belief in me and for their constant support and friendship.

I also want to thank Ardelle's son Jon Danks for first proposing this book; Ardelle's daughter Julie for her encouragement; my son Zachrey for his guidance through the foreign world of computers, disk drives, and data bases; my son Marshall and his wife, Jodi, for their long-distance support of this project; my daughter Clair and my friend Kasey Shantz for their editing advice; my attorney Kingsley Holman for his legal counsel; and my many friends who have taken delight in watching me fulfill a dream.

I want to acknowledge *Mpls/St. Paul Magazine* for publishing my story, "The Dark Side of the Heart," in 1987. It encapsulated my family's experience in Ardelle's transplant and laid the groundwork for this book.

I also want to acknowledge the publishers who have guided me when I needed it and encouraged me always. Specifically, I want to thank David Wexler, Donna Hoel, and George Cleveland, whose interest in the subject inspired me.

My final tribute is to the people who have been willing to share their experiences and knowledge with me. I hope that I've accurately reflected their honesty, their joys and frustrations, and their legacy of experience from which all of us can learn. I am deeply indebted to each of them.

Pat Stave Helmberger

Transplants: Unwrapping the Second Gift of Life

INTRODUCTION

This journey began when my sister Ardelle learned she had amyloidosis—a rare and mysterious disease. Strange deposits were settling in her heart, leaving her exhausted, short of breath, swollen, and extremely ill. Eventually Ardelle's heart had to be replaced. And so we began moving into a whole new world of organ transplantation.

I have put my thoughts together not only as a tribute to my sister's courage but also in the hope others out there might be helped. I learned nearly all organ recipients share the same hopes, fears, side effects, and joys of renewed life. Nearly all donor families share the stunned disbelief of sudden death and the healing consolation in giving life to a stranger. And most professional staff who work with both recipient and donor families are touched by the pain and share in the joys that are inextricably linked with transplantation.

I've attempted to be as honest as possible in my exploration of this subject. As a journalist, I set out to look at transplant issues from a human interest point of view. This is not an account of a medical procedure but rather an account of how people respond when faced with life and death decisions and how those decisions affect them.

During a year and a half, I've spoken with organ recipients and their families, donor families, and medical personnel. I've explored the psychological and emotional price each has paid, and I've looked at the ethical issues involved in this expanding field. I've agonized over the financial stresses many recipients face.

This is not a public relations book for any person or any medical procedure or facility. It includes both praise and criticism. But as I look back on the hours I spent at kitchen tables, in restaurants, and in hotel rooms listening to the stories of recipients, I can tell you that, in nearly every account, I found an overwhelming sense of gratitude toward those who made the difference between life and death.

Each of the stories in this book unfolds through the words of the person or families involved. As new insights opened for me, I added "Guideposts" after some stories. These remind us of some of the complicated issues growing out of the receiving or giving of the gift of life.

By far the most difficult conversations were those I had with donor families—difficult because the pain is still with them despite the passing of time. As we peeled away the layers of emotion, I often found anger and resentment. And as I listened, I realized that the key issues of brain death and donor family support needed to be addressed. But in spite of what some donor families see as an inadequate system, most of them found consolation in having given life through death.

As I spoke with medical personnel around the nation, I found dedication and determination to unravel some of the mysteries that still confront this new area of medicine. They are asking questions such as how can we more effectively help recipients and their families deal with this major event? Can we discuss more openly the sexual issues involved? How can we better serve donor families?

Introduction

These are questions that plague not only the medical staff but the recipients and donor families as well. Many of them had suggestions for increasing the effectiveness of the program. The individuals are, I believe, the people best able to articulate their own needs. And those needs seem to be as much emotional and psychological as physical.

My goal is to look at the human side of this historic procedure and offer insights from those who have gone through it. If any of those insights bring understanding and comfort to even a few, I will consider that an inestimable reward.

P.S.H.

Transplants: Unwrapping the Second Gift of Life

Prologue

Ardelle: Where the Journey Begins

When my sisters and I grew up in Lengby, a small town in the woods of northern Minnesota, life was simple. Eight of us lived in a crackerbox house with an old radio as our only connection with the world. We had no running water and no well. Rain barrels caught our water for baths and laundry, and we carried pails of drinking water from a neighbor's well. We heated our home and cooked our meals with wood stoves, and we sat in the outhouse with spiders in summer and snowdrifts in winter.

We went to the Norwegian Lutheran Church—never to the Swedish Lutheran Church. Somewhere along the way I learned that God was a stern taskmaster with a giant blackboard in the sky, keeping track of good and bad deeds. The Devil stood by, waiting to skewer us on his pitchfork and toast us like marshmallows over eternal flames.

When our two older brothers went to war in their bell-bottomed trousers, we were sure they were the bravest sailors in the U.S. Navy. My sisters and I planted victory gardens and listened to our mother cry when reports of battles reached us. During those years, our mother and father managed first a grocery store, then a restaurant. Our sister Ardelle, nine years older than my twin sisters and ten years older than I, became our caretaker.

Ardelle cooked, washed dishes, and ironed our puffed-sleeve cotton dresses. When she was done for the day, she would gather the three of us around her and, in the glow of a single light bulb, read us stories and poetry. Sometimes we turned the radio on, and she would teach us to dance the two-step and the waltz to the sound of country music.

Our grandmother, who lived across the road in a haunted house, would sometimes take care of us when Ardelle had a date. From the cocoon of her feather bed, she told us ghost stories that filled us with terror. There were tales of the giant rabbit possessed by the restless spirit of Grandma's dead brother, the spirit of her husband's first wife, who removed the diamond earrings from Grandma's ears, and the ghost of her dead son, who visited her in the early evening hours when she was alone.

Darkness terrified us. After an evening with Grandma, the three of us little girls often crawled into Ardelle's bed and huddled against her for comfort. At our urging, she placed knives in the attic door so no ghost could get out, or she turned on the flashlight to be sure the scraping at the window was a tree branch and not a lost soul.

In our little village, babies were born and old people died without much ado. There were no doctors in our town. On the rare occasion that one of us was sick, my father, who never owned a car, hired a neighbor to drive us to a town seven miles away. Once I smeared my face with poison ivy so I could go for that ride. It worked—except by the time my parents decided I should go to a doctor my eyes were swollen shut and I couldn't see the sights of the town.

Prologue

Medical miracles didn't happen, and no one expected they would. People died of diabetes, heart attacks, and cancer. There was little preventive medical care except for the vaccines we lined up in the little brick school house to receive.

My grandmother believed in preventing illness by wearing copper wrist bands, placing raw potatoes and large leaves on her body, and drinking pink clover tea for its healing power. If a heart transplant had ever been discussed as science fiction, she would have, no doubt, stomped off, denouncing it as the devil's work.

Indeed, the heart has been considered the center of love, hate, compassion, anger, and bravery. Ballads, poems, novels, plays, and films have enlarged on that symbolism. It should be no surprise, either, that many heart transplant patients suffer more from depression and anxiety than other organ transplant recipients. Psychologists believe, because of the myths surrounding the heart, there is more fear that such a transplant could change the recipient. Myths die hard; in fact, some never die.

Other organ transplants, such as kidney, liver, bone marrow, and lung, don't carry the same misconceptions. We think of those body parts as what they are. We don't see any of them on Valentine cards, revere them on religious icons, or hear them celebrated in songs and poems. They are not endowed with emotions and intelligence.

Superstitions of the heart need to be put aside as outdated, along with Grandma's ghosts. The most potent symbol of love will undoubtedly remain the heart, but we need to remind ourselves that the brain does the loving,

15

though it's not likely we'll ever see it on Valentines or anniversary cards.

Since our childhood, my family has seen great changes in life and the world. Grandma and our parents have died, and the crackerbox house is gone. The radio that once linked us with the world is now a conversation piece in my sister's home. Car phones, computers, and satellites intimately connect our shrinking sphere. As a nation we've reached the moon and the space beyond and have left our debris among the planets. And we've found new and wonderful ways to live.

Medical science has created a bridge between life and death with organ transplants. Through years of struggle and experimentation, medical experts have found new medicines to curtail organ rejection and have implemented a computerized system of coordination to help connect donors and recipients. Now it's possible for a patient in need of a lung to receive a heart and lung and donate his or her own heart to another person.

My sister and thousands of others have had their lives extended because medical science has outgrown the past and because donor families are wise enough to give life in death. The gift becomes reality through the network of people who make it so: the donors and their families, the medical personnel, the organ transplant communication system, and the recipients and their families.

But the gift doesn't come without a price tag. It is not so much a miracle as it is a complicated extension of our will to live. We are willing to travel into unknown terrain, into an uncertain future, simply because life is precious. The people I've written about in this book are a testimony to that indisputable truth.

It is my hope that, for others who must travel that same terrain, this book will offer insights to the journey and hope for the future.

Transplants: Unwrapping the Second Gift of Life

1

Ardelle: A Change of Heart

Ardelle loved Christmas. It was a time for her to bake and knit and keep in touch with her family and friends. She sent her hand-fashioned scarves, mittens, and bedroom slippers off in many directions from her home in Fairbanks, Alaska, each wrapped with a special flair. She always kept Christmas cookies and Scandinavian delicacies on hand for visitors, and packages piled up under the tree with each shopping trip she made. There was something childlike in her excitement about putting up the tree and placing each decoration just so. And she felt a little sad when all of it was over and the tree and the decorations were put away. But she always had another project to begin.

Ardelle worked hard all her married life, helping her husband build houses in Alaska and tramping through the wilderness to hunt and pick berries. A veteran of 30 Alaska winters, she faced the long dark months when the moose stood stomach-deep in snow in her back yard, and she loved the brief, bright summers when the sun dipped below the horizon just before midnight.

She raised her children there, and when her marriage ended in 1982, she stayed—held, she admitted, by what poet Robert Service described as "the spell of the Yukon." There were the dogsled races, the city-wide betting on when the ice would go out on the Nenana River, and the camaraderie among people who face nature's harshness together. There was the ice-fog that made ghosts of people and houses and chopped sounds into brittle pieces. There was the Matanuska Valley where crops grew twice as fast and twice as big under the Midnight Sun as they did anywhere else, and there were the rivers where on a warm Sunday afternoon you could still pan for gold.

She lost her home and most of her possessions in a summer flood and was awakened on occasion by the rumblings of earthquakes. Once when she was on a berry-picking excursion, a bear accosted her and her husband on a mountain trail. Her husband, with their small daughter on his shoulders, sent a bullet through its brain. It fell, growling, a few feet from where they stood. Alaska is not for the faint-hearted. But for the adventurer with a pioneer soul, it's magic.

I understood Alaska's magic because, when I was twenty-one, I spent a year with Ardelle and fell in love with it, too. But I didn't have my sister's rugged spirit, and I came back home to Minnesota before a second long winter took hold.

In 1986 my family and I were shocked to learn that our pioneering sister wasn't well. She called our sister Marilyn one day in mid-January to let her know that she had seen a Fairbanks doctor. It seems that right after Christmas, Ardelle began to notice increasing exhaustion and breathing difficulties as well as swelling in her feet and ankles.

"I thought I had just overdone Christmas, you know, baking a lot and wrapping presents. I was always on my feet. But the doctor says I have a heart condition. Me, who's never sick! If I don't feel better soon, I'll go down to Anchorage and see a heart specialist," Ardelle said.

She didn't improve, and in March she made the trip by plane to Anchorage. She learned she had a rare disease called amyloidosis—a word that meant nothing to any of us—and it was killing her by depositing insoluable material into the tissues of her heart. She had three to six months to live, the doctor explained, because there is no cure for this mysterious killer.

Ardelle was managing a Fairbanks gift shop at the time, but the effort of going to work on the bus and spending the days keeping shelves stocked and waiting on customers became too difficult. She gave up her job and stayed at home. She tried to help with her grandchildren but found even that was too difficult.

By mid-May taking just a few steps exhausted her. My sisters and I begged her to come to Minnesota for another medical opinion. We knew we faced some great odds: Ardelle had little money and no health insurance. But we knew we lived in a state that was unsurpassed in medical skill and access.

I was working then at the First Unitarian Society in Minneapolis where a retired physician served as chaplain. I went to him and asked for advice. He said, "There's only one thing to do under those conditions. Take her to the emergency ward of Hennepin County Medical Center (HCMC). They won't turn her away. Doctors are always interested in rare diseases, and amyloidosis is rare."

Next I called a suburban legislator to get his advice. It was the same: "Take her to Hennepin County Medical Center."

I called our twin sisters Marilyn and Marion and told them what I had learned. They agreed we'd have to take her to HCMC, but we decided we should make an appointment at the University of Minnesota Hospitals as well. Marilyn made the arrangements and we kept in touch with Ardelle by phone until she set the time of her arrival in the Twin Cities. It was a Tuesday in early June when we three sisters and Marilyn's husband, Peter, waited nervously at the airport for the plane to arrive.

We were shocked when we saw Ardelle roll down the concourse in a wheelchair. Her normally pink complexion was sallow and gray and her feet were badly swollen. She had lost a great deal of weight and could take only a few steps without gasping for breath. As she struggled into the car and fell back against the seat, I realized just how sick she really was. I felt cold with fear that we might not be able to find the help she needed.

She had gone through an awful ordeal already, flying alone from Fairbanks to Seattle and from Seattle to Minneapolis with no one who knew how ill she was. At the time, of course, we didn't fully comprehend the desperate state of her health, either.

We drove to Marilyn and Peter's home and sat and talked and laughed as we always had. But the twins and I stole glances at each other that expressed our wordless concern and fear.

In the morning I went back to Marilyn's house. Ardelle was very ill—struggling for breath and swollen with accumulating fluid. Marilyn had gone to work and Marion and I decided we had to get Ardelle to the hospital right away. We helped her to the car and drove to HCMC.

I was terrified that they might just give her some pills and send us home.

We struggled in the door, Marion and I on either side of her. "My sister is very sick," I told the receptionist. "We need help for her right away."

Ardelle's pallor confirmed my words, and the receptionist called a nurse to come to the desk. After attempting to find a pulse and blood pressure with little success, the staff whisked Ardelle into the emergency room. Marion and I were close behind.

Doctors converged, ordered equipment, connected Ardelle to a heart monitor and oxygen, and prescribed heart-regulating medicine. In the midst of the activity, Marion and I slipped out to call Marilyn who worked nearby. Within minutes she was there.

And within minutes Ardelle was taken to the Cardiac Intensive Care Unit where Dr. Charles Herzog examined her further. Then he met with the three of us.

"Your sister is dying. Her only hope is a heart transplant," he said. "I'll get in touch with the university right away and see about getting her on the transplant list."

We were stunned. "Oh, my God!" Marion exclaimed, looking at Marilyn and me in astonishment. Our faces, no doubt, reflected our shock, in return.

"But she doesn't have any health insurance," I blurted.

"There's no better state to be in than Minnesota when it comes to health care," Dr. Herzog said. "I'll get in touch with David Conradi-Jones here at the hospital, and he'll help you through the paperwork for medical assistance. Ardelle will have to declare that she is now a Minnesota resident but under the circumstances, that shouldn't be too difficult. She'll never get back to Alaska without a transplant."

The next day I was with Ardelle when Dr. Herzog returned to see her. He hadn't yet mentioned the transplant possibility to her, and my sisters and I were afraid that she might say no. We had talked to her children by telephone the previous evening, and her son Jon believed she would never consent to go through it.

"Ardelle," the doctor began, "the amyloid has nearly destroyed your heart, and I can offer you only one chance at life. That's a heart transplant. Is that anything you'd consider?"

"No," was her quick response.

I watched her smooth the sheets with slow, deliberate motions—a gesture I had seen my mother make when she was dying of cancer. I reached for Ardelle's hand to make her stop. "Please, just listen to him before you say no," I pleaded.

"I've talked to the university, and they'd like to see you. Two of the doctors will come over and just explain the process to you. We've got some insurance details to work out, and then you'd have to go through some tests to see if you can get on the list. You'd be only the second person in the world with amyloidosis to have a heart transplant. But we know that the first person is doing well two years after surgery," Dr. Herzog explained.

"It wouldn't hurt to just talk to them," I encouraged.

"I'm too old," she said. She was fifty-nine, and very close to the cut-off age for transplants in 1986.

"Let them decide that," I urged.

"Well, I suppose I could see them," she said, still with a note of hesitation in her voice.

"Good," Dr. Herzog said. "I'll let them know."

After he left, Ardelle and I sat quietly together. It takes time to absorb the idea that, after having made some uneasy peace with mortality, another person's heart could offer life. We knew nothing of the process and had only heard of transplants on TV and in the newspaper as things that happened to people we would never know. Now the possibility had just been handed to Ardelle.

I called the twins when I got home to let them know Dr. Herzog had talked with Ardelle about a transplant. "She doesn't seem very enthusiastic," I told them.

"It's a major step," Marilyn said. "It's going to take some time to think about. Just meeting the doctors from the university is a start."

I agreed. As I called my brothers, Darrell in Brainerd, Minnesota, and Bud in South Dakota, to let them know what was happening, I thought about the thing we call "the will to live." It's what drives us through the myriad problems life deals us. In spite of grief and loss, physical pain, and economic woes, life is precious and worth living. I hoped Ardelle was thinking about her children and grandchildren. I knew they would be her inspiration to take this giant step.

In the hope she would consent to a transplant, Ardelle and I met with David Conradi-Jones, a county social worker, who began the paper work for medical assistance. He established Ardelle's residency and financial and medical need. He then hand-delivered the papers so the state approval board could review them the next day. We couldn't believe how quickly and effectively he overcame major obstacles.

Every day my sisters and I went to see Ardelle. Our brothers came as often as they could to buoy her spirits. And each day we watched the heart monitor anxiously and talked with the staff. They gave us the "no frills" truth; with each passing day Ardelle grew weaker and her heart more erratic.

Two weeks after Ardelle was admitted, Marilyn got a call from a staff doctor. Ardelle was failing, and a new medicine had been administered. "You had better tell her children to come right away if they want to see their mother alive," the doctor told Marilyn.

When the twins and I arrived at the hospital, we found Ardelle on a respirator and in a coma. We stood around the bed, holding her hands and talking to her, but there was no response. Our hopes of a transplant seemed now like a dream. I looked at this small, silent figure who had been part of my life since I was born, and my mind raced back to memories of childhood.

One of my most vivid memories is of the four of us girls huddled on the sagging daybed with Ardelle reading from a tattered book of poetry. "Little Orphan Annie," "The Village Blacksmith," and "The Wreck of the Hesperus" were filled with magic for me. I owe her my lifelong love of poetry for it was she who introduced its rhythms and emotions to me.

I was nine years old when I began writing my own verses, sitting in the crook of my grandmother's tree. My poetic attempts improved as I grew up, and at fifteen I sold my first poem. Not many years ago, Ardelle called me from Fairbanks and said, "Guess what? I just saw one of your poems in a newspaper I happened to pick up. That really made my day!" As I stood by her bed, all those memories converged in me and spilled over in tears.

Ardelle's son Jon arrived that evening from Anchorage and he, too, was overcome with grief. "Mom," he said. "It's Jon. I'm here." But there was no response. He laid his head against hers and wept. Late that night we left the hospital exhausted and sad. We needed sleep to endure the next day.

When tomorrow came, we found Ardelle improved. The doctors explained that a bad reaction to the new drug they were using to stabilize her heart had caused the setback. She was still on the respirator, but she was awake and able to write messages and nod her head. Giddy with relief, we began to hope again.

Our hope intensified the next week when the university doctors came to talk with Ardelle about a transplant. "The tests are rough and take about a week," they told her. Because of her disease, she would need a kidney biopsy and a bone-marrow test in addition to the standard blood, lung, dental, eye, and gynecological exams. Then there was the "soundness of mind" test. Marion and I were with Ardelle when the psychologist came in to administer it.

"You can stay," the psychologist quipped, "but no coaching."

We promised, and he began with questions such as what city are we in? What hospital is this? Who are the president and vice president of the United States? What is the total of 15 plus 25, 71 minus 50?

When he was finished, he got up and shook Ardelle's hand. "You get an A plus," he said proudly. "And good luck to you, Ardelle." Then he was gone and the tests were completed. Now another wait began until the university doctors made their final determination.

July arrived hot and humid. Ardelle's daughter, Julie, came from Fairbanks with her five-year-old daughter Samara. That was a highpoint for Ardelle, and she wanted to celebrate the Fourth of July with a traditional picnic. Dr. Herzog agreed that a trip into the open air would be a boost for Ardelle's mental health. One of the nurses helped us move her out on the balcony, high above the city. We ate fried chicken, potato salad, and watermelon. The heat was stifling and, to me, oppressive, but Ardelle was thrilled in spite of the assorted equipment that sat beside her.

On July 8, Ardelle's sixtieth birthday, we decided to throw another party. The hospital staff, who by that time had become part of the family, thought it was a great idea. We decorated the room with streamers and balloons and ordered a white cake with fresh strawberries. Marion and Marilyn had given Ardelle a soft white robe as an early gift so she could wear it at the party. Marion curled and combed her hair and painted her long nails. She looked like a young woman half her age as she positioned herself against the pillows like a queen on her throne.

Brothers, cousins, nephews, nieces, and friends arrived bearing gifts. Staff members stopped in when they could take a minute from their duties, and even Dr. Herzog came in for cake and strawberries. He had become the symbol of hope for our family and Ardelle's guardian angel. Her eyes sparkled as she sat beside him for a picture before he had to dash off.

When the other guests were gone, the twins and I picked up the discarded plates and wrapping paper and put the room back in order. Ardelle was getting tired, even though, according to her, it was the best birthday party she'd ever had. "I suppose it's time for us to get going too," I said. "You could use a nap."

A knock on the door interrupted us. The door opened and a slender, dark-haired woman entered. She was Dr. Maria Teresa Olivari, a member of the University of Minnesota transplant team. She had a present, too—the news that Ardelle had passed all the tests, and with her consent, she would be placed on the transplant list.

"What a present," Marilyn said, putting her arms around Ardelle.

But Ardelle again seemed hesitant. "I'm sixty years old. Someone younger should be on the list instead of me."

"Let me explain things and then you can think about it," Dr. Olivari said gently. "You know, it might take up to two months to get the right heart. It has to match your blood type and be the right size. Most donor hearts come from young people in motorcycle or auto accidents who are brain dead but have a functioning heart. Once a suitable donor is found, surgery takes place within a few hours. The transplant itself is the simple part; it's the aftercare that's most difficult."

She told us that after surgery, Ardelle would be placed in isolation because the anti-rejection drugs suppress the immune system and infection is a major concern. Usually a patient stays in the hospital for about two weeks and then goes home with lots of medication and a transplant manual in which to record all the medication intake. The manual includes a list of side effects the medicine can cause.

"We will be monitoring your health through biopsies and blood tests, so you'll be seeing a lot of us afterward. You'll need to maintain a proper diet and exercise program, too. It's not easy and it's a lifelong commitment, but it's life," she said.

She talked to us about the myths of the heart, too, and how we've invested it with love and hate and reverent feelings. "It's just a pump, but sometimes people think that a change of heart can mean a change of personality. Of course that isn't so."

We were enthralled with the possibility of life she offered and, as I recall now, we asked very few questions. I remember thinking that everything was suddenly speeding up, and I wanted to say, "Stop!" But I knew that every passing day diminished Ardelle's chances to live.

"Now it's up to you, Ardelle," Dr. Olivari said. "Here's my card with my number on it. Call and let me know what you decide. I have a feeling I'll see you again because I think you'll say yes." With that, she bid us good-night and left, closing the door behind her.

The four of us huddled closer together. We knew the risk of saying no, but the risk of saying yes was like orbiting the moon: There's a dark side and a light side and we'd have to go full circle. And although the family could support Ardelle's decision, one way or the other, it was ultimately hers.

We separated quietly that night, and as I walked to my car, I felt a closeness to my sisters that both comforted and frightened me. I was sure we took our sisterly relationships for granted because we'd always known we could count on each other for help and understanding. If suddenly one of us was gone, that small, intense circle would be broken. What impact that break would have I could only guess.

But in less than a week Ardelle had made her decision. The twins and I walked into her room one evening and found her, as usual, reading a book. She closed it, marking her place slowly. Then she smiled an impish smile and said, "Well, I called Dr. Olivari today."

"You did?" Marion said. "And what did you say?"

"I said I'd go for it," Ardelle replied.

"Oh, that's great," I exclaimed, "That's just great!"

She laughed. "I told Dr. Herzog I didn't dare say no. You three would probably kill me if I did!"

We were especially joyful that evening with renewed faith that, after all, this could have a happy ending. And we stayed later than we should have, talking and giggling like school girls.

For the first few days all of us were on a high, full of anticipation and hope. But I soon discovered I was not prepared for the trauma of waiting for someone else to die so that Ardelle could live.

One afternoon as I drove home from work, I heard an ambulance siren, and I began to wonder if someone young and healthy had been critically injured. I wondered if that heart might be the one to save my sister's life. It was as if my values had gone awry and accidents were good and brain-injured teenagers were the answers to prayers. It was just a fleeting thought that mid-July day, and I didn't say anything about it to anyone.

A few days later as Marion and I drove down the highway, we passed a young motorcyclist without a helmet. "Gee," Marion said. "I wonder what blood type he has."

"Oh, God, you think about that too!" I said, feeling a sense of relief that I wasn't alone in doing so.

"I know it's awful," she said, "but I can't help it. I've always thought I was a fairly good person, and here I am waiting for someone to die."

With each passing day and every malfunction of Ardelle's dying heart, the thought of another person's death intensified, as did my ghoulish interest in accidents and ambulances. Finally I called my friend, Barbara Amram, a social worker and counselor.

I explained what was happening and said, "We're all beginning to feel like vultures hovering over a death scene."

"I can imagine that's exactly how you feel. It sounds like you're taking on guilt for a death that hasn't even happened, one you have no control over and certainly won't be responsible for," she said. She assured me that this reaction was common among people who know their loved one can live only through the death of someone else's loved one.

That conversation helped me, and although the thoughts persisted, I didn't feel quite as criminal as I had. My sisters and I began to talk more openly about our thoughts, and that helped, too. I wish now we had had some warning about these feelings.

We coped as best we could and made our daily trips to see Ardelle, who was growing weary of hospital life in spite of all the visitors, flowers, and cards. That sweet, brief day in the sun on the Fourth of July now seemed a long time ago. She begged to go home to Marilyn and Peter's house, even for a weekend.

Dr. Herzog, concerned about her psychological health, agreed to a change of scene. She would have to remain on a heart monitor and an alarm system, and Marilyn, Peter and I would have to be trained to use the equipment. It wasn't terribly complicated, but the machines looked menacing. Peter, a police officer trained in CPR, wasn't as nervous as Marilyn and I. After two sessions, Dr. Herzog said Ardelle could go home on July 25, less than a week away.

On July 20, two days before my birthday, a few friends had a surprise party for me at my home. We lounged on the floor, relaxing with some wine, and I told them about my apprehension of those awful machines. "I just know I'll panic and push the wrong button or something," I laughed.

The phone rang and I got up to answer it. It was Marilyn. "Pat, the hospital just called. They've got a heart for Ardelle, and we have to go down right away and transfer her to the university!"

"I'll be there in a few minutes!" I gasped.

I hung up and started laughing and crying: "They've got a heart! They've got a heart!" I threw my arms around my friends and they cheered and hugged me back.

"Oh, I've got to unplug the coffee pot and feed the cats and. . . .I've got to get going!"

One of my friends put his hands on my shoulders and said, "I'll drive you. I don't think you're in any shape to drive yourself." I looked down at my trembling hands and agreed.

When Marilyn, Peter, and I arrived at the hospital, Ardelle was sitting in a wheelchair, calm and smiling. The staff, bubbling with joy, hugged and kissed her as we said good-bye and wheeled her downstairs to the waiting ambulance. I rode beside her while Marilyn and Peter followed in the car. It took only a few minutes to reach the university. Then began a long night.

The staff drew vials and vials of blood and ran tests to be sure the match was perfect. There were papers to sign and a myriad of white-smocked people coming and going. Marilyn called Marion, who had briefly gone home to Phoenix, and I called Ardelle's children to let them know the good news. Sometime after midnight Peter went home to get some rest while Marilyn and I stayed at the hospital.

At some point in that eventful night, Dr. Ring, a transplant surgeon, came in to tell us that the match looked good and the donor team was on its way to retrieve the heart. Surgery would begin sometime the next morning.

Marilyn and I knew we had a long day ahead of us, so shortly before dawn we went to the family waiting room to rest. Sleep was impossible—there were too many thoughts racing through my mind. I felt intense joy and deep grief. I knew that while we looked forward to the miracle of tomorrow, there was another family facing the shock and grief of an unexpected death. I wanted to hug them and thank them, but that was impossible. We were nameless strangers giving and accepting a priceless gift.

As I twisted and turned on the small sofa, I felt we were going headlong into an experience we knew nothing about. As part of society's first transplant generation, we were without a chart or a compass. We had nothing to do but trust a host of people we'd never met. The surgeons, the donor team, the helicopter pilot, the lab technicians—each of them had a vital role in saving my sister's life.

At eight o'clock Marilyn and I folded our blankets and went to see Ardelle, who had not gotten much sleep either. An hour later we accompanied Ardelle to the door of the operating room where we kissed her and squeezed her hands. I remember feeling terribly inadequate as a comforter, without words to express my fear, hope, and excitement.

"I'll see you later," she said as she disappeared behind the door.

As if it were an ordinary day, Marilyn said, "Well, let's go have coffee."

So began our wait. During the long morning, family members came and went. We made phone calls and walked the corridors. The morning passed.

At noon Marion arrived from Phoenix. We had more coffee and waited for word of Ardelle. Two o'clock came and we still had no word. Finally at three o'clock, a surgery liaison came to talk with us.

"There's been a complication and the donor heart hasn't arrived yet. It's on its way now by helicopter and should be here any minute," she said.

I turned instinctively to the window and scanned the sky. I felt as if I had suddenly stepped out of myself, and it was another woman who stood by the window, watching for a helicopter bearing a human heart.

Fifteen minutes later, the helicopter arrived and the heart transplant took place without complications. By six o'clock the operation was over, and two surgeons came to tell us the good news. After an initial false start, the heart was beating strong and smooth. Exhausted but elated, we went for more coffee to give us one last boost before we went to visit Ardelle in her isolation unit. We could only see her briefly before we went home for some much-needed rest.

When we arrived at the isolation unit and looked in the window, we were stunned by the assortment of tubes and machines that surrounded the bed. Ardelle was barely visible in the midst of the equipment. Marilyn and Marion put on the sterilized clothing necessary to enter, and I burst out laughing. Each only 4-feet, 11- inches tall, the twins were swallowed up in the hospital garb, their hands and feet lost. But after some folding and tucking of excess fabric, they rustled through the door. Peter and I watched through the window as they touched Ardelle and talked to her. She lay very still, eyes closed, attached to tubes and ventilator, the heart monitor measuring every beat of her new heart.

I felt suddenly overcome with emotion as the scene through the window unfolded like a silent movie. I turned to Peter, tears streaming down my face, and collapsed into his arms. "I just can't go in there," I sobbed. "I just can't do it."

"That's okay," he whispered. "You can do it tomorrow. We all need to go home and get some sleep."

The next day was July 22, my birthday. Refreshed from sleep and a shower, I entered Ardelle's isolation room clothed in gown and mask. I admit to being intimidated by all the equipment, but I found Ardelle's hand and squeezed.

"It's my birthday, Ardelle, and I got what I wanted," I said.

Although her eyes were still closed, she squeezed my hand in return and I knew she had heard me. My tears were hot and sticky behind my mask.

Guidepost: Living with the Guilt

One of the most troubling aspects of the transplant procedure is the wait for an organ. Many of us who have waited believe the medical community should better prepare us for this emotional event, unlike any other that human beings have faced.

As one spouse told me, "We need to be forewarned about the guilt often associated with waiting and hoping for an organ. We know someone will have to die—and it's usually a young person and a sudden death. If we could just talk about it and share it, it wouldn't seem so awful. Counselors should spend some time with the families just letting them know this might happen."

Ardelle suggested counselors should be organ recipients themselves. "Only they would understand the issues we face every day and how our lives are changed," she said. Another recipient agreed. "This is something you can't understand unless you've been through it. It's like having a recovering alcoholic counseling alcoholics. There's a connection that's a vital part of the treatment."

Bill: Love Takes a Detour

Bill Holden received his new heart on July 26, 1986, five days after Ardelle's transplant. It was the day Bill and Sondra Smalley had chosen as their wedding date. Five months later when they finally spoke their marriage vows, the heart of a 16-year-old accident victim from Mandan, North Dakota, was beating in Bill's chest.

Bill, a slender six-foot, six-inch Yankee from Massachusetts, had open heart surgery in 1979, suffered a heart failure in 1981, and lived on drugs for five years until 1986. A Unitarian Universalist minister and superintendent of a juvenile reform schools program, Bill kept a busy, demanding schedule and refused to accept his physical limitations. When a transplant was first suggested to him at the age of 52, he was shocked but reluctantly agreed to an evaluation. He passed the tests and was placed on the waiting list for a heart.

Bill and Sondra Smalley, a psychologist credited with coining the term "co-dependency," met in 1984. Despite Bill's deteriorating health, they set their wedding date.

"Everything was done," Sondra said. "The church, the reception—it was all in place. I had chosen a red and yellow dress and our friends had planted a field of red and yellow zinnias for us. Then suddenly his health declined drastically and we canceled the wedding."

Bill could no longer live alone and care for himself, so he moved in with Sondra. Her son, Doug, helped to literally carry Bill up and down the stairs. In nine days' time Bill became so ill that Sondra rushed him to a hospital where he remained in intensive care for 31 days. On each of those days doctors told Sondra that Bill's death was imminent.

Doctors were pessimistic about finding a heart for him because of his unusually large size and high antibody count, a result of his previous heart surgery.

Sondra stayed with Bill every day, feeling certain that it would be his last. His children and sister came from Vermont. Friends arrived from Florida. Her own life was "on hold," along with his. Her work as a psychologist was suffering, and the physical and mental stress left her exhausted. One evening, after getting home from the hospital, she planted flowers by flashlight. "Just to get my hands dirty, to do something normal," she said.

The strain of mourning and hoping at the same time took its toll. "We have no models about how to do both simultaneously," she said. "I would think one minute, 'My God, he's dying' and the next minute, 'No, he'll get a heart.' How do you mourn with a smiling face? I'd wish for someone to die and then feel guilty because I knew we weren't waiting for a 95-year-old person to die. It had to be a healthy young person."

Then the call came that a possible match had been found. Bill was moved to the university for tests. But the heart wasn't right for him, and it was given to someone else. He returned to his hospital bed, disappointed and deeply depressed. Three other possible matches failed, too, and the couple's dreams crumbled further with the loss of each precious opportunity.

Bill was kept sedated by morphine and knew only bits and pieces of what was going on around him. He remembers the day, however, when, as a drastic measure to prolong his life, doctors prescribed 1,000 fluid ounces of water each day. "I knew enough about medicine to understand that death was very near," he said.

He floated in and out of consciousness and pain, euphoria, and depression. Two days before the transplant, he told Sondra, "I can't go on. Do I have your permission to give up?"

She took his hand and looked at his haggard, pain-ridden face and whispered, "Yes, Bill." She pressed her face to his and felt his tears mixed with her own.

As they parted that evening, she was certain they had said their final good-byes. Sondra drove home and fell exhausted into bed, sleeping and waking, expecting the hospital to call with the news of Bill's death. But the phone didn't ring.

In the morning she went to the hospital and found him amazingly better, watching Prince Andrew's wedding on television. The see-saw of hope and mourning took over again. She spent the day with him, but he could see the strain in her face.

"Go home and rest, honey," he said. "If I get a heart you're going to need strength to go through it with me."

Late that same evening he called Sondra and said, "Something's going on. They're taking blood samples."

Sondra called the nurses' station and asked what was happening.

"Yes," one of the nurses said, "we are doing tests. They'll run them all night and by morning we should know whether or not there's a match."

"How will we know?" Sondra asked.

"The university will call when they know for sure, but they don't want to move him in his condition unless the heart is definitely right," the nurse told her.

Sondra sat up all night waiting for the call. Finally it came.

"It's a match, Sondra, and Bill's on his way here now," the doctor told her.

"I'll be there as soon as I can!"

The drive seemed to take forever, and every stoplight seemed permanently red. But the doctors weren't happy when she finally reached the university hospital. Bill had an infection and fever.

"If we can't bring the fever down, we can't do the surgery," the doctors told Sondra.

But two hours later, his temperature was normal and surgery was on. Sondra held his hand and kissed him.

"I'll see you, honey," he murmured as he disappeared behind the sterile white operating room doors.

Sondra, elated and grateful, called two close friends to join her at a near-by hotel for a glass of champagne. It was time to celebrate. She knew that Bill was safer than he had been for years.

In the midst of the celebration, however, Sondra was suddenly struck by the reality of what had happened. Someone young and healthy had died. A family somewhere was in shock and grief, and they had given Sondra and Bill the only wedding present that mattered at all.

Four hours later when surgery was completed, she donned the sterile gown, booties, gloves, and mask and entered the isolation room where Bill lay entangled in tubes and machines. He was struggling to free himself, and Sondra and the nurse had to hold his arms still so that he couldn't loosen or remove the myriad tubes inserted in his body.

Bill was alive but he continued to suffer.

The week following surgery he developed a painful bladder infection. And because his prolonged hospitalization had caused his muscles to atrophy, he needed physical therapy to build them up. Then there was the constant monitoring for organ rejection. His recovery was slow, and after the first high, he slipped again into a deep depression.

"I had made my peace with death and now I was alive. I had to adjust to life again. The world gets very small when you're dying, and you tend to withdraw from those you love. You're letting go. And then, when you get the transplant, you have to take hold again. That takes time.

"My mind wasn't functioning very well and neither was my body. I couldn't remember my medical procedures and I had no strength. Sondra had to learn all about my medication schedule before I could go home."

When he finally was released from the hospital, Bill found life hadn't changed much for either him or Sondra. He still needed to be dragged up the stairs, and his mind was still fuzzy.

"I wanted to be useful," he said, "but it would take me all day to make a grocery list and get the groceries. I couldn't lift my feet up the curb, so I'd have to struggle to the handicapped access to get into the store. I couldn't lift the bags, so someone always had to be there to help this six-foot-six guy carry a few groceries.

"People see depression in transplant patients as ingratitude. There are so many expectations people have of you because you've gone through a medical miracle, and you can't feel the way they expect you to feel—alive, full of vigor, born again, renewed. You're struggling with drug reactions, additional diseases, diets. I couldn't remember anything and I could hardly walk. It took me about three years to get over the depression.

"For the first two years I asked myself if it was really worth it. One of our friends even said to Sondra, 'Bill has no gratitude.'

"He was right. I didn't. I had developed drug-induced diabetes. I was getting fat, with puffy cheeks and a prednisone pregnancy, as we call our extended stomachs. And you always have to worry about getting sick because the medicine suppresses the immune system and any little germ can do you in. I was depressed, and there was very little psychological support from the hospital staff. They were so busy keeping us alive that they didn't think about how we lived. I was grieving for the way life used to be when I was healthy, but I didn't know it. I was grieving for my slender face and my flat stomach.

"I was wrapped up in my own symptoms and the medication regimen, and I didn't have time to think about Sondra and what it was all doing to her. When you're sick, people have significance only for what they can do for you."

It was wearing on Sondra. She was trying to get her business re-established at the same time that she was driving Bill back and forth for the host of medical examinations and biopsies, then going to the pharmacy to pick up the antirejection drugs. Still she maintained their home and worked in her garden.

Each time the doctors gave permission for Bill to take on a new responsibility, Sondra stopped doing it for him. He started to drive and take care of his own medical schedule and drug intake. Sondra knew from her professional experience that chronically ill people do best when they are treated normally and, although Bill sometimes didn't like it, he took on an increasing amount of responsibility for his own care.

After the first three-month rejection period had passed, they rescheduled their wedding for December 20.

The wedding was held at a beautiful French hotel near Minneapolis. Their families and friends gathered to celebrate not only a wedding, but a renewed life and the sustaining love of friends. Instead of the red and yellow dress she had chosen for her summer wedding, Sondra wore a street-length navy silk. She stood beside her beloved Bill, and they spoke the words that officially made them husband and wife.

"Everybody cried," Sondra remembered. "And everybody we invited came, and nobody wanted to leave. It was a beautiful wedding."

They went to Key West for their honeymoon, along with all the medicine. Sondra drove the rented cars and carried the bags and worried about Bill. When they returned to the Minnesota winter, life continued to center around medicine and doctor's appointments.

"There isn't much talk about life after the transplant. There's just the glamour of the actual surgery. We don't talk about the stress that significant others go through, and they often become the invisible person whose own emotional and physical needs are ignored. And that can't go on forever without serious consequences. Divorce rates are high among transplants," Bill said.

Bill and Sondra remember the March afternoon that her pent-up emotions exploded. He was worrying about another symptom that was developing and Sondra had what she termed a *tolerance break*.

"In other words, I got mad. I yelled at him, 'I don't want to hear about another symptom. I'm pissed. I'm mad. I don't want to hear about one more medicine! I've had enough, enough, enough!'"

Bill was deeply hurt, but he got the message that Sondra's stress level had definitely peaked.

"I'd been like a zombie for months," she said. "I didn't have a lot of time for feelings. I just got mad that day and it was long overdue. I wasn't mad at Bill. I was mad at life. You can't live forever on the original high of the transplant. There's so much responsibility, so many demands. With something as dramatic as a heart transplant, the recipient gets a lot of attention, and everybody wants to hear the story. It takes over every conversation, every social occasion, and I didn't want to hear it anymore. Life goes on."

Gradually Bill began to look for other support so Sondra could get away from it awhile.

"What saved my life," Bill said, "was hearing from an earlier transplant patient that things get better. That was all I needed to know. But I needed someone with credibility to tell me that.

"I started to look for ways I could feel useful, but I was still very limited in strength. I decided to volunteer as a chaplain for the St. Paul Police Department. That helped me to begin thinking about other people and how I could help them, and I started to feel worthwhile again.

"I remember one night, though, when I was pretty nervous. I went with the police to a domestic violence situation, and the police left me there to talk to the violent partner. I was still as weak as a kitten, and I knew I couldn't protect myself if he got violent again, so I just sat and talked and talked until he fell asleep."

Bill made other changes in his life, too. As superintendent of the juvenile reform schools, he had held a managerial position. After returning to work, he found he preferred direct contact with the youth and their families. He also found it was easier for him to display his feelings.

"I received so much love in dying that I wanted to give some in return. Now I'm called the hugging minister and I don't mind it at all," Bill said.

Two years after the transplant he did something he'd been thinking about for a long time. He wrote a letter to his donor family. It was a warm and grateful tribute to their gift of life that came to him and Sondra on a very special day. He has not received acknowledgment of the letter, but the Red Cross assures him the family received it. For Bill and Sondra that was the important part.

In the process of healing, he's had to redefine what's normal for him.

"I never used to have to get up at night to go to the bathroom. Now it's normal for me to get up three or four times a night. Another thing that's normal for transplants are wicked, wicked muscle cramps. You have to learn to stretch and work them out.

"It's also normal for many male transplants to be impotent, but nobody wants to talk about it. So much of the male ego is wrapped up in sexual virility. When a man is impotent, he doesn't want to be reminded of it, so he pushes away his partner and that may contribute to the high divorce rate. We need to have some research done on it, and we need to learn new ways, besides just copulation, to find sexual pleasure."

Bill believes that Sondra's strength and honesty provided the support he needed to find his own strength again and to allow both of them to get on with their lives. He's at work full time and Sondra's business is flourishing, but they still take vacations in England and Hawaii.

"We've discovered," Sondra said, "that life is for living. We plan for the future and live in the present."

Both the present and the future contain the medicine, the check-ups, and the dietary restrictions all transplants live with. To de-emphasize his "prednisone pregnancy," Sondra has helped Bill put together a carefully selected wardrobe.

"He was always so slim that he didn't have to worry about hiding his tummy. Now he wears navy or charcoal sweater vests that detract from the bulge, and he stays away from plaids or prints," she said.

They've also designed and built a new home that incorporates both their private and professional lives. Still there's room for children and gardens. It's a home of dreams and hope and a symbol that life is on course again after the very long detour they had to make.

Guidepost: Learning to Cope

As Bill Holden said, most of the general public hear only the glitz of transplants and know little about life afterward. The answer to most of the difficulties recipients and family members go through is simple, yet difficult: It's communication.

"We need counseling," Bill told me one day on the phone. "There has to be more recognition of the grieving process that some of us go through. That's part of the depression people think is ingratitude. Many of us grieve for our past lives, our past appearance, our past lifestyle. It's wonderful to be alive but in many ways, we're very different. It's almost as if you can look down the path and see the person you once were. And you have to wave good-bye and maybe shed a few tears while you do it," he said.

More counseling is also needed about impotence in male transplant recipients. Most of the people I visited with talked openly about the stress it has brought to their lives and their marriages. Yet, in many transplant programs, it remains a mystery shrouded in secrecy, like an elephant in the middle of the living room that no one admits is there. But for the average male, impotence is devastating. It can bring deep conflict to a relationship.

A heart recipient explained just how devastating it can be. "If I had known I wouldn't be able to perform sexually, I might have said no to the transplant. But nobody told me. For most men, a job and sex are life's greatest motivators. After my transplant, I lost my job *and* my sexual ability. That's pretty rough to go through."

Another explained that recipients need counseling to find ways other than intercourse to enjoy sexual pleasure. "But," he said, "it's a subject that's basically ignored, and it affects our quality of life and our relationships." He speculated that impotence and other stress factors may be responsible for a number of divorces among transplant couples.

When I first met a 48-year-old heart recipient, I asked, "What one suggestion would you make to medical personnel for improving the program?" His immediate response was, "Find out why many of us are impotent."

I set out to ask that question of doctors and psychologists involved in organ transplant programs. Two of the surgeons believed it was psychological. One explained it this way: "By the time people come to us to talk about a transplant, their marriage is often already in tatters because of a prolonged illness. There's a lot of dependence by the male, and that doesn't do much for the ego. Most of them aren't on medication that should produce that effect."

When I talked with a transplant psychologist at the same facility, his answer was quite different. "I think it may be the result of heavy doses of medication. You can't put all those pills into one body and not expect some changes, including impotence."

I asked another doctor how a patient could give informed consent to a transplant if the possibility of impotence isn't explained. "That's a tough choice. We don't know what causes it, and if we tell them it might occur, the power of suggestion may make it more likely," he said.

"But you're not talking about it and it's still happening. So the power of suggestion can't be part of the problem," I said.

I wasn't finding any definitive answers to my questions and the mystery intensified when I received the results of a study on sexual function after transplantation published in the December 1989 *Journal of Heart and Lung Transplantation.* It had been conducted by Thomas Mulligan, MD, Helen Sheehan, BSN, and Josephine Hanrahan, BS, at the Medical College of Virginia and the McGuire Department of Veterans Affairs Medical Center in Richmond, Virginia.

A survey of 115 male heart recipients with a mean age of 47.9 years (24 to 64 years), with 62 percent of them responding to the survey, showed the following:

- 92 percent had an available sexual partner, with 74 percent married and living with their spouse.

- Mean time since transplantation was 28 months (range, 30 to 80 months).
- Each patient took an average of 8.4 different medications daily, mostly cardiovascular and blood pressure drugs.

These men perceived themselves to be in "fair" health, with 93 percent reporting some form of daily exercise. Few reported feelings of hopelessness or worthlessness. In general, the study indicated, libido was strong and remained unchanged after transplant.

In contrast, there was a persistent impairment and gradual decline of erectile rigidity and orgasmic ability. About 80 percent perceived the gap between libido and sexual ability to be a problem, and they reported an interest in undergoing evaluation and treatment if available.

The study also found that those who perceived themselves to be in "good" or "very good" health were more likely to have strong libido. An earlier study by Dr. Mulligan reflected the same information. It indicated that a person who perceived himself to be in poor health had a sixfold increased risk of being sexually dysfunctional.

Researchers had expected to find erectile function and orgasmic ability improved after transplantation. Instead, they discovered erectile function was only "sometimes adequate for intercourse" before and deteriorated further at three months and still further at one year after transplantation. This trend, they found, was consistent among respondents.

Intercourse after transplantation was relatively infrequent, taking place approximately once per month, compared with published reports of 1.5 times per week for healthy middle-aged men. Intercourse frequency was related to both patient and partner libido, before and after transplantation, but was most closely related to erectile rigidity. The study found no significant relationship to exercise tolerance, immunosuppressive protocol, specific classes of drugs, or number of drugs.

While researchers believe their study makes an important contribution to the subject of impotence, they indicate it may have certain weaknesses. For instance, only a male veteran population was surveyed; they would have preferred a higher response rate than their 62 percent; and they admit to a relatively small sample size. Still, it is one of the first descriptive surveys done on an issue they believe is vital to the quality of life, and they encourage further research into post-transplant impotence.

That's exactly what most heart recipients want, too. They want to know if it's physical or psychological or a combination of both, and they want to know what can be done to help them. They want researchers to keep asking the questions even if the answers seem elusive now. The elephant in the living room needs to be acknowledged.

Transplants: Unwrapping the Second Gift of Life

3

Ardelle: Homecoming

Ardelle's recovery was blessedly uneventful, and she and Marilyn began the process of learning the medical regimen in anticipation of her release from the hospital. They had to study the transplant manual and record the numerous pills and liquid drugs needed each day. They had to make appointments for the following week, practice using the blood pressure gauge, and learn about what to eat and how to exercise.

At home, Marilyn cleaned Ardelle's room until it sparkled and brightened it even more with fresh flowers. The entire family was on hand for the excitement of her homecoming on a hot August afternoon. Ardelle settled in a lounge chair on the patio while we toasted her with champagne. Marion agreed to stay for a month to help with the medication and doctors' appointments while Marilyn was at work. Their world revolved around the bottles and boxes that contained Ardelle's life-sustaining medicine. The twins made excellent nurses, fulfilling Ardelle's every wish.

It seemed that every time I went to see her, she was eating. The medicine gave her a voracious appetite, and food became her major concern. She weighed less than 100 pounds when she had the transplant, but by mid-September she had gained 10 pounds. Her cheeks began to take on the roundness that goes with the medication.

All of us began coming down from the high. I worked every day and, as a single parent, took care of my family, my home, and my yard. As the fall drifted into winter, I went less often to see my sisters. Marion returned to Phoenix, and Marilyn and Peter took on most of the responsibility for Ardelle's welfare.

It's always easier to see things from a distance, and as I look back, I know I failed to carry my share. I didn't fully comprehend the pressure Marilyn felt. Not only did she help with the medical regimen, but she also had a growing concern that Ardelle didn't always follow her diet or get the necessary exercise. Both Marilyn and I felt Ardelle was depressed: She slept late, read, and watched lots of TV. She often didn't get dressed, and she rarely talked about her feelings.

With very little understanding of what life after a transplant is like, or what psychological effect the medications can have, we began to feel angry. It didn't appear Ardelle was happy with her second chance at life.

We knew she was becoming increasingly frustrated with her appearance. She had always been slim and attractive, and now her body was thickening, her slender face was puffed, and her joints ached. Buying a new wardrobe wasn't fun because the sizes were bigger and the cuts were chosen to cover her "prednisone pregnancy." She was apprehensive about seeing people because they often made thoughtless comments about her looks or, as she said, "they stare at my chest and I feel like a freak. I know they're thinking about me having somebody else's heart."

Christmas came, and Ardelle was rejuvenated. She decorated Marilyn's house and baked and shopped. She sent boxes of gifts to her children and grandchildren in Alaska and cards to her friends around the country. And she admitted she missed her family and Alaska.

It was time for her to think about going back, although the medical complications of changing residence were major concerns. However, the University of Minnesota and the State of Alaska worked out the details of her care. In late summer of 1987, Ardelle boarded a plane to make a journey we once thought she could never make.

The next year, Ardelle's son and daughter both moved from Fairbanks, Alaska. Her son went to Seattle and her daughter to California. Ardelle went along, making her home in California, too. Photos showed she was losing weight and enjoying the rambunctious antics of grandchildren. Her life was getting back to normal. Her brush with death had given all of us a new appreciation of each other and a new devotion to the small, often overlooked joys of life.

In our happiness we tended to forget the deadly disease that still lived in Ardelle's body. Little did we dream that in four and a half years it would once more begin its deadly work inside Ardelle's new, vibrant heart.

Transplants: Unwrapping the Second Gift of Life

4

Betty and Wesley:
Trading Up

"Is your dad getting our mom's heart?" were the first words spoken between the two families sitting in the waiting room at the University of Minnesota Hospital on December 11, 1989.

Betty Youness was about to become one of the first live-heart donors at the University, something she had offered to do when she was accepted on the heart/lung transplant list. She needed healthy lungs to replace hers, which were badly damaged by the genetic disease Alpha-1 anti-trypsin enzyme deficiency.

After two and a half years of waiting, she received the heart and lungs of a donor from the Kansas City area, and her heart went to Wesley Olson of St. Paul.

Betty was 35 years old when her illness was initially diagnosed in 1977. She was first hospitalized in 1982, and entered the hospital again in 1985. In December 1986, she read a news article that said a world-renowned heart/lung surgeon at the University of Minnesota Hospitals was going to begin doing transplants on people with her disease. Excited, Betty made an appointment. Six months later, after participating in a medical regimen to build her strength, she passed the required tests and was placed on the waiting list.

As she waited, doctors prescribed oxygen to ease her struggle to breathe. She was losing weight and energy. The usual household chores were too much for her, and grocery shopping was out of the question. She could do a few loads of laundry if the humidity was low, but climbing stairs completely sapped her strength.

Lori, Jean, and Dan, Betty's children, took over much of the housework, but when they didn't do it the way Betty wanted it done, she let them know. Life went on as normally as possible, and Betty's husband, Larry, and her son Dan continued their weekend hunting and fishing trips to the family cabin.

The family wore what 18-year-old daughter Jean described as "a mask." Everybody was positive and everybody avoided dealing with the fact that Betty was dying. Larry focused on the prospect of a transplant, knowing there was nothing else that could save her. Betty's determination to live gave him hope.

In a touching description of her feelings, Jean said she shied away from close relationships. "I didn't want people to get to know me and then feel sorry for me. I didn't want to feel dependent on others. Maybe deep down I didn't want to get close to people because that might mean losing them in the future—I don't know. Stress had been a large part of my life, and I coped with it in many different ways. One of the ways was to withdraw from my family. Nobody ever tried to talk about my mom's illness, it was just too hard to discuss."

Jean slept a lot in the afternoons, and her eating habits were sporadic. She'd starve and then binge. When she was in sixth grade, Jean was bulimic and spent many days at home, sick. Her studying was as irregular as her eating. Weeks would go by without her doing any homework. Then she would dive into it to forget about her mother's illness.

In the evenings, the family played cribbage, played with the family dog, Chester, and watched television.

"I laughed a lot," Betty said, "and I enjoyed my life most of the time. I didn't want to talk about my illness because whenever I had a bad episode of coughing the kids would get so frightened. So we just went on day by day, doing the best we could."

At the same time, Betty suffered from depression masked as irritableness. She tended to get upset and angry.

"I'm an 'up' person usually, but there were times when I got down. I began to wonder if I'd ever get my transplant because I'd waited so long and not even one call had come from the hospital."

The myths of the heart didn't play a role in Betty's transplant because she thought of herself as getting lungs, not a heart. Afterward, she tried not to think about what actually happened in that operating room.

"I've seen hunting pictures," she said. "And I know they actually opened my chest and took out those organs, and I was virtually dead for a while except for those machines. It's just amazing what was done."

Wesley Olson was amazed, too, when he learned that he would receive a live donor's heart. His own had caused him problems since 1980 when he first went into cardiac arrest. He, his wife Lorna, and Lorna's sister-in-law were driving in St. Paul when Wesley blacked out.

"Wes," Lorna had cried, "you're going through a red light!"

But Wes didn't answer. He had slumped over. Somehow they stopped the car and Lorna's sister-in-law jumped out and ran for help.

When the paramedics arrived, they laid Wes out in the street and shocked his heart three times before it began to beat regularly. He stayed in the hospital for three weeks and then had heart by-pass surgery on December 15. By February 1981 he was back at work.

Then, one evening when Lorna was out, he decided to go watch their son play hockey. It was probably a wise decision because when he went into another cardiac arrest there were lots of people around to call the paramedics, who once again revived him. After a few days rest, he went back to work.

For the next seven years, with the exception of minor medical interruptions, life went on as normal for Wes, until one afternoon when he went to fill his car with gas at a station a few blocks from home.

"After leaving the station, I began to feel that something wasn't quite right, so I quick turned the wheel of the car and that's the last thing I remember. I woke up and my car was on somebody's lawn. I sat there and I didn't know what had happened. The next thing I knew I was sitting in the kitchen telling Lorna I didn't feel good. I drove the car home and I don't even remember doing it," he said.

Lorna called the paramedics and they took him to the

hospital, where he remained for a few days until his heart once again was stabilized.

Wes's doctor told him there wasn't anything she could do for him, but she referred him to another clinic. He stayed there for a month and underwent extensive tests. After he was discharged, he went back to work for a week, but another heart problem landed him back in the hospital. It was July 7, his and Lorna's thirty-third wedding anniversary.

It was during that hospital stay that he learned his heart had deteriorated to the point where only a transplant could keep him alive. The tests showed that his heart speeded up to 250 beats per minute, causing him to lose consciousness. His heart wasn't really pumping at that rate, it was simply quivering.

He went to the University of Minnesota for an evaluation and on September 7, 1989, he was accepted on the heart-transplant waiting list. He was unaware that Betty Youness had already been waiting for a new lung for over two years.

Through the long summer of 1988, Betty's 22-year-old daughter, Lori, drove her to the transplant support group at the university. Lori got to know and love many of the other people who were, like her mother, waiting for organs. Heart/lung patients, she learned, wait longer for transplants and their levels of frustration seemed to increase with each passing day. The group decided to bring their need to the public and undertook to promote donor awareness. Nevertheless, several of them died before organs ever became available. Lori was grief-stricken. This experience, the pressure of waiting for donor organs, and her mother's declining health further exacerbated Lori's emotional turmoil.

On August third, Larry and Betty planned a quiet dinner out to celebrate their twenty-fifth wedding anniversary. That morning as Betty read the newspaper, her spirits were dashed. Dr. Jamieson, her hope for a transplant, was leaving the university. To Betty it felt like the death knell.

"We went out that night, but the joy was gone and I was really depressed. I pouted through most of the evening," she said.

The news hit the family hard and Lori's depression deepened as others on the waiting list died. One day, during the support session, Lori's emotions finally gave way.

"She had taken on a lot of the responsibility for donor awareness publicity," Betty related. "And she began to apologize to everyone for the lack of donor organs. People were shocked at what she was saying, but they all realized what was happening. She was treated by a psychiatrist and she seemed to get better. Then she and my sister, Diane, went to Atlanta to the United Network of Organ Sharing headquarters to better understand how the system works. She seemed to feel better when they returned, but by the next fall, she became ill again. Most young people don't experience these kinds of losses, and she didn't let me know how she was feeling because she thought it would make me worse.

"The second time she got sick, we called the Crisis Intervention Center when she began hallucinating. She wanted to go and get help."

Lori was hospitalized for two weeks, struggling with fear and depression. She finally overcame them. Lori came to learn that in her role as eldest daughter and main caregiver to her mother, she was putting her own feelings on hold for her mother's sake.

During those stressful days, Lori and her family continued to hope with each ring of the phone that the critical call would come and Betty's life would be spared.

Then, on December 11, at 7:20 in the evening, someone from the university called.

"We own a small business," Betty recalled, "and December usually means Larry works late. So that night I was fixing pancakes and eggs. I hadn't eaten yet because I was doing the cooking. Jean answered the phone and recognized the caller as a transplant nurse. She handed me the phone and I finally heard the words I had waited so long to hear."

"We have a donor for you, Betty. Of course, you can turn it down if you choose," the nurse said.

"Turn it down!" Betty exclaimed. "No, I've been waiting for two and a half years for this!"

"Have you eaten yet?" the nurse asked.

"No, " Betty answered. "I was just about to sit down."

"Feed it to the dog," the nurse said.

Betty balanced the two eggs she had just cooked onto the spatula and flipped them into Chester's dish. Then she began to clear the table.

"Try to be here by eight o'clock," the nurse said.

"We put the milk in the refrigerator and one of the girls canceled a date," Betty remembered. "Then we all got in the car and drove off. I don't know what other people were thinking or feeling, but I was sad leaving home. I didn't know if I'd be coming back. And driving over the Lafayette

Bridge—it was so beautiful. The doctor had told me that one of the complications of a transplant is death. That came back to me as we drove to the hospital."

Earlier that same evening, Wesley Olson had gone Christmas shopping with his son. His other son stayed home with his mom.

"Don't forget your beeper," Lorna had cautioned before Wesley left.

But he forgot it anyway. Fortunately, Wesley walked in the door ten minutes before the hospital called. Then the race was on.

There was little time for either patient to think once they arrived at the hospital. Tests began, and Betty underwent ultrasound to be positive her heart was still in good enough condition to donate. It was.

Betty was told that the recipient of her heart had arrived at the hospital. In their separate rooms, they were each prepared for the medical procedure that would turn their lives around. Soon Betty Youness and Wesley Olson, who had never met each other, would be lying in adjoining operating rooms, participating in a drama that had begun with the death of a stranger far away.

When the surgeries began, at three in the morning, the families of these two found themselves face-to-face in the hospital waiting room, having a conversation unparalleled in history.

"It was strange," Larry remembered. "We overheard these people talking about their father getting a heart, and Lori just walked over and said, 'Is you dad getting our mom's heart?' After we discovered he was, nobody knew what to say."

Wesley's surgery was completed first and both families went to see him. The Youness family waved to him through the isolation unit window. Betty's surgery was finished at noon.

The doctors kept Betty in an induced coma, wanting as little motion from her as possible. Twice she was returned to surgery and was packed in ice immediately afterward. Jean remembers that Betty's head was wrapped in towels and there was blood on the floor of the isolation room.

"She was kind of purple and yellow," Jean said. "My sister Lori and I would go in to talk to her. We'd say, 'Mom, you're gonna be okay. You don't look too great, but you're gonna be okay.' She'd squeeze our hands, so we felt that she heard us."

One day Lori went in to visit the man who had her mother's heart. She beamed down at him and whispered, "You're my Mr. Mom."

"That endeared her to all of us," Wesley said.

Betty's parents came to see Wes, too, telling him that they had nine daughters and had lost their only son, but now they would claim him as theirs.

Betty regained consciousness on Christmas Day, nearly two weeks following the transplant, after a long and difficult struggle for life.

Christmas and New Year's came and went and both families postponed their celebrations until Betty and Wesley could go home. Wesley went home on January 2 to celebrate both his January 4 birthday and his belated holidays, but Betty remained in the hospital.

Betty's birthday was January 3 and she celebrated it quietly with her family. She watched the January snowfalls and the early descent of winter darkness from her hospital room as the days dragged on.

One afternoon, a stranger walked in to her room.

"I looked up at this guy I'd never seen before and saw that he had tears in his eyes. I knew right away it was Wesley. I reached out my hand to him and asked, 'How's my old ticker going?' That was the beginning of a friendship that will last a lifetime, I'm sure," Betty said.

On the first of February, Betty went home. She breathed deeply of the crisp winter air without the aid of an oxygen tube, feeling that the year's new beginning symbolized her own. On Valentine's Day, an appropriate day to celebrate love and life, Betty and her family gathered for their belated holiday festivities.

"We decorated a big plant in the living room and put the presents around it. We had had more time to shop," Jean said, "and we got in on all the sales."

Betty received a special-diet recipe book and a tennis racket and balls, wrapped in silver foil to remind her that she had promised Dr. Jamieson she'd learn the game when she was well again. Betty gave each of her children little bags of heart-shaped candy.

But, after a few weeks of near euphoria, Betty experienced depression and found herself crying for no apparent reason. After a few more weeks, her sunny nature took over again and life at the Youness' house became brighter than it had been since 1977, when Betty first learned of her disease.

Wesley's recuperation was uneventful. Although he was thin—he weighed 112 pounds—and his muscles had deteriorated, he didn't suffer any depression or mood swings. Lorna didn't pamper him or allow the boys to do so.

"I learned as a young person just how destructive that can be," Lorna said. "When I was 14 I had polio and was partially paralyzed. It was an awful time for my family and me. I was so depressed that I thought about suicide a lot. When I saw someone walk by me, I would cry for hours because I couldn't walk. I was really feeling sorry for myself.

"Then my parents took me to a Camp Kuwanis and just dropped me off. I said I didn't want to stay, but they said, 'We'll see you next weekend,' and they left. That week made me see myself and my life in a different light. I began to realize that I was able to do a lot of things, and I began to feel lucky that I was only partially paralyzed. So many kids were in much worse situations than I was.

"I've carried that lesson with me all my life, and I applied it to Wesley. There were times when I felt very sorry for him, but I never let him know. When he first came home from the hospital, I set out his medication, because it's pretty complicated. But after a couple weeks, I said, 'Okay, it's all yours now.' And of course he took over right away."

Both Wes and Lorna believe that by receiving the heart of a live donor they were spared the mixed feelings of those who receive an organ through death.

"It just made it much, much easier," Lorna said.

Betty and Wesley have attended some of the clinic sessions together.

"People would say, 'Oh, there's Betty Youness. She gave her heart to that guy who's with her.' But I wasn't thinking that way. He certainly doesn't owe me anything," Betty said.

Wesley had a hard time convincing people that he now has the heart of a woman who is alive and well: "Some people still ask me, 'Wes, is that really true?' I can understand them not believing me. I find it pretty amazing myself."

Betty is indeed alive and well and she watches her family with pride. She sees her son, Dan, changing since the transplant and is convinced that the stress of her illness repressed the real Dan. He's begun dating, buying new clothes, lifting weights, and going out with friends. Her daughters, too, are able to lead their own lives.

Lori is in her own apartment now, and Jean is developing friendships and doing well both socially and scholastically.

Betty has written three letters to the donor family but hasn't mailed any of them.

"It's a difficult thing to do. I assume I'm writing to the parents of a young adult, and with kids of my own, it doesn't come easily. I know I had nothing to do with that death, and my name wasn't even mentioned. It didn't come into the picture until they had given permission for the organs to be removed. It's just trying to say thanks for being so generous at that awful time, and trying to say it with some decency. I don't want to overpower them with how wonderful it is to be alive because their person is gone. It's very hard for me to put it into words. It would be easier for me to talk face-to-face with them."

Betty has gained 35 pounds and has the puffy cheeks that go with the medicine. The medicine also creates a ravenous appetite and when she's alone, she tends to nibble.

"I never had to worry about my weight because my disease controlled it. I needed more calories just to breathe. Now I have to think about losing those pounds," Betty said.

Her new-found freedom is still exhilarating for her. Even grocery shopping or driving to her cooking class at the hospital is fun.

"I think that people who are sick for a long time, as I was, really appreciate being well again. And I think that families who see their loved one deteriorate over a long period of time have a different attitude, too, than families whose loved one is sick for just a short time," Betty said.

The medication regimen, often something transplant recipients complain about, doesn't bother her. She's taking less now than she was before the surgery.

"What's a handful of pills twice a day when now I can walk to my pharmacy to pick them up!" she said.

In July 1990, Betty was one of the people who carried the Olympic Festival Torch through the Twin Cities.

"She ran only a little way, but we were all so excited about it," Jean said.

Wesley wasn't in that festival, but he wishes he had been.

"It would have been so great if Betty could have passed the torch to me just as she did her heart," he said.

Guidepost: Being Aware of Family Needs

In order to shed some light on the issue of family stress in transplantation, I called my close friend, Barbara Amram, who had helped me through the uncharted waters of Ardelle's transplant journey.

Barb is a school social worker who was selected in 1988 as Minnesota School Social Worker of the Year. She's spent 25 years working with parents and children and conducting adult communication classes.

But beyond her professional qualifications, I trust her compassionate, no-nonsense approach to life. And as the mother of a son with a physical disability, she's lived through most of the problems I wanted to talk with her about.

First, I asked her to explain the psychological needs of a family going through the stress of a critical illness, especially when young children are involved.

The basic needs of children, she said, are nurturance, emotional connectedness, and reassurance of acceptance and love. "In growing up, children have many dependency needs that are fulfilled by parents—and adolescence, one of the most volatile periods in a child's growth, is no exception.

"It's about this time they're beginning to realize they aren't immortal. That's complicated by having to deal with the mortality of a parent who's sick enough to need an organ transplant," Barb said.

I explained to her that two families I had spoken with said it was too difficult for them to talk with their children about the possibility of death if an organ didn't arrive in time. Everyone knew the family members were critically ill, yet they simply avoided the subject. "Can you tell me why this happens? I asked.

She nodded. "Yes, I can. It's called denial, and it's one of the defenses we use when the odds are so tremendous, as in this situation. Perhaps it reflects the fact the adults haven't accepted what's going on. Before a parent can comfortably talk about death with a child, they must have come to some level of acceptance. I'm not saying total acceptance. I'm not sure there ever is such a thing," she said.

"How could these families be helped?" I asked.

"First, you'd have to help the adults through that stage. Then they could be more receptive to discussing it with the children at their level.

"Young children can't always understand the intricacies of surgery and waiting for a heart transplant. But they can understand what the realistic level of hope is and what the doctors can do to help. Parents may be able to help the children by admitting to their own stress and fears and then encouraging the children to talk about theirs.

"Parents can't change the situation. They have no control over what is going to happen. But what they can control is how they deal with it and how the children can talk about it and share their feelings. The anxiety level may be diminished somewhat if a child can feel that it's okay to be scared and nobody's going to be angry about that. In a home where it's not being talked about, the kids don't know what's safe to say, but you can count on the fact they understand a lot more of what's going on than we given them credit for.

"The whole transplant scene is a difficult one to deal with. When you add the complication that a person can live only if an organ is found, the stress levels increase. There's always the chance that an organ won't be found in time. If you had a parent with cancer you might give as optimistic an opinion as possible about the chances of survival with different forms of treatment. But that's different from having it hinge on the additional unknown of whether that organ is going to be available. Teenagers can understand what's happening, and it's important to discuss it with them. To keep it a secret may make things worse. Frequently a person's fantasies are worse than the reality of the situation," she said.

"How could a parent's chronic illness interfere with a child's development?" I asked her.

"Perhaps the worse-case scenario," she said, "would be if a child 'got stuck' at the level of development he or she was at when the parent becomes ill. Let's say the child was six years old, and life up to that time wasn't too bad. Now this terrible thing has happened. It would be more comfortable to revert back to behavior characteristic of a younger child. That would be a very serious response. Short of that, many other things could happen. The child could become depressed, overwhelmed with guilt, or feel abandoned. He or she could develop phobias or begin acting out. Kids need someone to talk to, whether it's a friend, a cousin, an aunt, or anyone they feel close to.

"The child could also be affected by the financial problems that usually surface in these situations. For instance, does the family have its basic needs met of food, clothing, and shelter? Those things are essential. But beyond that, if the kids like to go skiing, they may have to give that up. If they're used to going out on Friday night, that may have to end. Their social development and independence might suffer," she said.

Barb believes there is little emotional support for families going through any kind of crisis, whether its handicapped kids or parents with serious physical or mental problems.

"I've talked with families who have these problems, and they tell me the medical field takes little interest in the emotional needs of families. I think it's a long-term failure of the medical profession not to recognize there are emotional needs and something can be done about them.

"The mental health aspect of a patient can't be overlooked. Almost always, the public has to be the advocate for services and changes in the law. Until there is an advocacy group that takes on the needs of a certain group of people, you're not likely to see much change. However, the family, when they're in the midst of the crisis, certainly can't rally around the cause. They can hardly deal with their own situation. It might take the survivors to begin to speak up about what would have helped them," she said.

"I certainly think a support group would be very helpful for those who are going through this. You're starting out with people who often have been very successful in their lives and who have very fine family communication and relationships. Now they're being put into an enormously stressful experience, and that's going to have an impact on the healthiest of people. Then, within the range of people being treated, there are going to be those who weren't as emotionally healthy to begin with. Those people may not be able to handle the stress, and it will tip the balance," she said.

"Is this problem the same in any kind of illness?" I asked.

"It's similar. But I think it has added dimensions in a transplant situation. The survival of a loved one depends on someone else dying. That's not something people have to deal with in other conditions. It strikes at a very basic value that all human beings are raised with: that life is good and living is good."

"During my research, I've heard about many marriage problems that seem to be related to the illness," I said. "Can you shed some light on that?"

She nodded. "Yes, I think I can. The family is a system and any change in the system affects its relationships. If you have a sick spouse, the role that person played in the system is going to be altered, whether as bread winner or chauffeur to Boy Scouts.

"That immediately puts more demands on the other spouse. That can mean doing the grocery shopping, the laundry, the cleaning, getting the oil changed in the car. Even if there was a good give-and-take between the spouses, things are still going to be different. Unless these people are very, very wealthy and can afford to have someone else do all the things the spouse did, someone in the family must do them.

"All of this will make the doer more tired, less patient, and sometimes resentful because this has happened to them. Some marriages can survive all of the above. Some become stronger. Sometimes they need professional help. Just being in this situation, they could use some assistance in dealing with the issues that naturally arise," she said.

"I guess what we've been talking about is communication," I said. "Parents talking to kids and to each other, not letting unspoken fears and stresses escalate into bigger problems. I think we're also talking about isolation, both individual and family isolation. Why is it so hard for people to talk to each other?"

"It's mainly fear," she said, "that keeps us silent. We're afraid of getting hurt and hurting others. We're afraid to show our weaknesses and our anger. We're afraid to show we don't have all the answers. And when you're talking about life and death issues, we're also afraid of upsetting the sick person because he or she might die. It's no wonder we don't talk. But we need to.

"The biggest irony of this whole thing is we don't take the emotional risk of exposing our feelings, but we're willing to take the huge risk of a heart transplant," she said.

Transplants: Unwrapping the Second Gift of Life

5

Connie: Facing the Fears, Celebrating the Joys

The church was filled with flowers, family, and friends. The bride, in a pink satin and lace dress, stood beside her beaming groom. Then to the strains of "Just You and I," they walked down the aisle together to begin a new and wonderful life. It was August 17, 1991, and she was becoming a wife and a step-mother of three sons whom she deeply loved. Ray, her groom, was the gentle, loving man she had longed for. Connie Hubbell-Eiden had accepted his proposal of marriage on the 18th anniversary of her kidney transplant—the date chosen specifically by Ray to honor Connie's commitment to life.

Connie's struggle for life began in the summer of 1960, when, at the age of 12, she developed Strep throat. Unlike most children, she didn't fully recover. She had no energy, her eyes grew puffy, and she passed blood in her urine. Her kidneys had been damaged by the disease glomerulonephritis, and doctors gave her the medical treatment available at the time: bedrest, cortisone, and blood pressure medication. As she grew stronger, she returned to school and got back into normal activities, closely monitored by her physician.

Transplants: Unwrapping the Second Gift of Life

In 1970, when she married a young man in the military, she was 24 years old and living a normal life. She moved with her husband to a military base in Calumet, Michigan. But that same year, her kidneys began to fail, and with the onslaught of menstrual problems, she grew anemic, requiring blood transfusions every few days. The poison that built up in her system brought nausea and an itch that was unstoppable. "I scratched myself until I bled. I would take a hair brush and rake my body with it. It drove me insane," she recalls.

The doctors in Michigan knew her condition was critical and transported her by plane to Wilford Hall Medical Center at Lackland Air Force Base in San Antonio, Texas, for dialysis while she awaited a transplant.

"When the plane left Michigan it was about 38 degrees, and when we landed in San Antonio, it was 110 on the tarmac. The plane was full of critically ill people, and some of us laid in the hospital lobby for two hours while they got us all processed in. Then they put me in a room with an elderly woman dying of cancer. The smell was awful. I was so scared. I knew I was dying, and then they put me in a room with death itself. They moved me out the next day, but it was a horrifying experience," she recalls.

"I wanted to talk to somebody about dying, but everyone danced around the issue. I was sitting there wanting to say, 'Shut up and listen to what I have to say because if I die here you're not going to be able to know what I want.' I wanted to discuss cremation and what should be done with the few good pieces of jewelry I had, and I was really angry that I couldn't even talk to my husband or mother about it.

"I felt at that point I had a husband who loved me. I'd been in 42 states. I had wonderful friends, and I was contented with my life. I wanted to tell people that. There were chaplains and psychiatrists I could talk to, but I wanted my family to listen and they didn't want to hear it," Connie said.

Then on November 12, 1972, an accident near the base took the life of a 19-year-old male. "The nurse came in and told me I might get one of the available kidneys and they would start dialysis in preparation," Connie said.

She was thrilled with the news and the hope of a renewed life. "I knew I'd live," she said. "I thought, 'With my guts and God's help, I'll be all right.'"

The surgery went without a hitch, and within a few hours the nurses walked her around the bed. Twenty-six hours later, she was no longer attached to any machines. She was euphoric for the first few days.

Then the depression set in. "Right after the transplant I was put on prednisone and immediately gained weight. You're sitting there with no neck and a face like a beach ball, and that's rough. By the time I left the hospital on December 16, I had gained nearly 30 pounds and was feeling as unattractive as I could possibly feel. I wore mu-muus and bedroom slippers.

"My husband had moved down to San Antonio by that time, and my mother came to stay with us for a few months. She and I went shopping at Penney's to find some clothes that would fit. Nothing looked right, and I started to cry and went back to the car. Mom put her arm around my shoulder and said, 'I saw some cute tops in the maternity section. Let's go back and see if we can find something there.' I agreed, and we found three cute tops that I wore over slacks with elastic waist bands, and they helped get me past the feeling that I was too frumpy to go out in public," Connie remembered.

"I had lost much of my interest in sex," she explained. "Food was a substitute. My husband and I went to the doctor to talk about it, and they laughed at us. I think they were embarrassed. But we were young people. I was 25, and he was 29. But I could go for six months and not care. I just wanted to eat."

Connie kept gaining weight because of the horrendous appetite the drugs created. "You felt like you could eat furniture," Connie exclaimed. "Okay, you've got a ham and a turkey here. I'll finish that—and if you have another one, I'll eat that, too. Nothing could ever put a cap on it. I weighed 181 pounds in a matter of a year or two.

"I tried a number of diets and joined Weight Watchers several times. The last time, it finally took, and I lost more than 50 pounds. Now I eat what I want, but I stay away from salty foods. I eat fish and chicken and a little beef. I don't drink alcohol, but I'm a great water drinker and usually have more than eight glasses a day," she said.

Despite her struggle with excess weight, the most severe side-effect of medication has been the mood swings. "I could go from being ridiculously euphoric to being furious because someone hung up a dish towel incorrectly.

"Then in 1978, when my marriage ended, my whole world was so bleak and I just wallowed in it. I thought about suicide several times.

"I've paid for this kidney in many ways. Not being able to have children was one. The doctors advised me against it because of the severe consequences it could have," Connie recalled.

But she survived those dark days, and with the decreasing amounts of medication, she began to feel she could lead a normal life again. She still has bouts of tears for no apparent reason and she gets angry quickly. "I want to throw things and bust stuff and really yell and howl—but then it's over," she said.

She bruises easily and in 1987 she bumped her leg on a desk. It developed into a blood clot that covered most of her lower left leg. "I wasn't able to go to work for almost six weeks, but I set up an office at home so I could continue working. I had to have a skin graft to repair the damage. I just didn't know if I could go through it. Every time you hit the wall, you wonder if this will be the time you don't bounce back," Connie said.

She weighed 181 pounds when she met Ray and she credits him with helping her lose her excess weight. They walked two or three miles three times a week. It was their opportunity to talk and share some quiet time together after helping his boys with homework and getting them settled for the night. "Even when it was bitterly cold, we'd bundle up and walk," she said. "I was losing about two pounds a week and was really feeling good about that."

Connie recalls that she didn't tell Ray about her transplant for several weeks after they met. "A doctor friend had said to me, 'Don't tell him. Wait until he figures out that you've got more energy and stuff going on than most people do.' I took that advice because I didn't know how educated he was about transplantation. When I finally told him, he just put his arms around me and kissed me. He said, 'I'm so glad it worked out right or I never would have found you.'

"He's with me all the way. He knows as much about my medication and condition as I do, and he encourages people to sign a donor card at every opportunity," she said.

Each year, Connie celebrates her transplant anniversary with a party. Last year her new family drew a picture of a large kidney with the state of Texas in the corner. It says in bright letters: "We Love You, Connie." That picture is center stage in the living room, as Bob, 12, and Greg, 15, lounge on the sofas with three sleepy cats.

Now tall and slender, Connie radiates joy. She is a testament to longevity, a high quality of life, and the supportive role of love. The love between her and Ray is predicated on mutual respect and trust, but in their wedding vows, they were more specific. She vowed her commitment "through thickening waistlines and fading eyesight," and he, in turn, promised "to comfort you when you're sick, to cheer you up when you're feeling down, to console you when you're in sorrow . . . ."

They've taken the reality of life and, by infusing it with love, they've continued its celebration.

Guidepost: Listening and Loving

Death is one subject most of us avoid discussing. But there are times when talking about it is an expression of love that we need to make. When Connie wanted to talk about it, no one wanted to hear her, simply because it was too painful.

I remember when my father-in-law was close to death, even though none of us knew it at that time. He was 86. One evening, while we were visiting him in the apartment that replaced his long-time home on the farm, he said to his son, "I don't think I'm going to live much longer."

"Oh, Pa," his son laughed, "you're going to live forever."

The old man reached his hand out to me and I saw tears in his eyes. "I just woke up one morning and I was old," he said. "It happened when I had to leave the farm."

As we sat side by side on the sofa, he reminisced about his sheep and the lambs he had to feed with baby bottles. He talked about the long walk to the river to go fishing and about snowdrifts so high he could tunnel through them to the barn.

We talked of happy times and pleasant family gatherings. It almost seemed as if we were summing up our friendship, capping it off with our shared memories. Within two weeks, he died. I have always treasured those hours we spent recalling the past. I think it helped him and I know it helped me.

Difficult though it may be, family members and friends need to make themselves available to listen when their loved ones need to express thoughts, fears, love, and memories. It validates life.

As Connie said, "I wanted them to know I'd had a wonderful life, but they didn't want to hear it."

Transplants: Unwrapping the Second Gift of Life

6

Mary: A Journey of Love

Although Mary Lund was the first woman in the world to receive an artificial heart, this is not a story about medical milestones. This is a love story about Mary and her husband, DuWayne, who wanted only to live their lives in peace, sheltered in the quiet countryside where life was sometimes harsh but always beautiful.

But one day in December 1985 Mary became sick with something very much like the flu, and within days she and DuWayne were catapulted into the spotlight. The world watched and waited as doctors replaced Mary's damaged heart with a mini-Jarvik artificial heart to keep her alive until a human heart was available.

The illness had begun, DuWayne said, on a Thursday. Mary left work at the Bethany Nursing Home early because she just wasn't feeling well. When DuWayne arrived home later that afternoon, Mary was in the kitchen thinking unenthusiastically about what to make for dinner. She wasn't hungry and spent the rest of the evening lying on the sofa watching TV.

On Friday morning she was no better and called in to work, saying she would see them Monday morning. By then she was sure she'd be fine. But through the weekend she became worse, vomiting even the water she tried to drink. She had the classic flu symptoms.

"I kept asking her if she wanted to go into town to see the doctor, but she said no," DuWayne recalled. "By Sunday night, she was so weak that she just laid in bed without moving. I called the doctor, and he wanted to talk to Mary. We didn't have a phone by the bed, so I helped her out to the kitchen. She sat on a stool at the counter with her head in her hands and answered the doctor's questions with yes and no. When she hung up, she said she'd wait until morning to go in when the clinic was open. I slept on the couch so I wouldn't disturb her, but about midnight I heard her call me. Her voice was so small and weak, and she told me it was time to go to the hospital.

"I started the car to get the heater going and made a bed in the back as best I could. Then I helped Mary get bundled up and we traveled the 15 miles to the hospital. Fortunately, the roads were clear and the snow made the night lighter. You know, when Mary and I first moved into our new home, she was afraid of the darkness. She had always lived in a city, and on our first night together in the house she asked me, 'Why is it so dark and so quiet?' After awhile she learned to love it and decided that she didn't want to live in the city again.

"The nurses and doctors were waiting for us when we pulled up to the emergency door. Dr. Stewart looked like he'd just climbed out of bed, and I felt kind of bad because I knew he had to work at the clinic the next morning. They loosened Mary's heavy robe and began taking her vital signs. Her blood pressure was extremely low, and she was dehydrated. The doctor said she'd be put in the Intensive Care Unit. 'She's very sick, DuWayne,' he told me. I said, 'I know she's very sick.' He repeated it again with the emphasis on the *very*.

"I sat in the waiting room for what seemed like forever, waiting for more information, but everybody was busy with Mary. About 7:30 A.M., I said I'd go home and make sure Mary's son, Scott, got off to school. Then I stopped by the shop and said I wouldn't be coming in to work.

"When I got back to the hospital, Dr. Stewart had called in a heart specialist. Mary's vital signs were dropping, and things didn't look good. He said I should get Scott and whoever else I wanted to be with me. I asked Mary's sister, Barb, to pick up Scott from school, and I called a few friends and asked them to come to the hospital. We sat without saying much. We were all stunned by the events of the past few hours.

"After a short wait, the doctor came in.

"'I'm sorry,' he said. 'Mary needs medical care that we're not able to give. She needs to be taken to Abbott Northwestern Hospital in Minneapolis where there's an excellent cardiovascular staff and equipment. There are no helicopters available now so we'll have to send her by ambulance.'

"Through all of this, I was in a state of denial. I wasn't facing the fact that Mary was critically ill. I just went along without fully comprehending. There wasn't room in the ambulance for me, so Scott and I were going to drive down. Before we left, the nurse accompanying Mary in the ambulance asked me for my license plate number and make and color of my car. I asked her why, and she said, "We might not make it there in time. She may die on the way. We'd have to notify you through the state patrol."

"The truth began to sink in. I suddenly understood just how sick she was, and I lost it right there, crying uncontrollably. I couldn't believe what was happening.

"After I got hold of myself, Scott and I rushed home and threw some stuff into a suitcase and headed for Minneapolis. The ambulance had gotten about an hour's head start, and I pushed that car as hard as I could. About 25 miles down the road we saw an ambulance heading back toward Alexandria. Scott and I looked at each other. We knew what that could mean. But I decided not to turn around. I figured if Mary had died they'd send the highway patrol after me, and if she was still alive we needed to keep going.

"I'd been at the hospital once or twice a long time ago, but I couldn't exactly remember where it was. As I drove toward Minneapolis, I began to see landmarks I recognized, and we got there without any trouble. It's a big place, but we found Mary right away. A team of doctors were working frantically to keep her alive, and nobody could give me any information. I called Mary's brother, Dick, and asked him to come to the hospital. He lived in Minneapolis, so he was there in a short time. Rev. Fred Booth from our church in Hoffman arrived, too. We were all in kind of a state of shock, and we couldn't imagine what had happened to Mary to bring her so close to death.

"Scott, Dick, and I just sat in the waiting room and waited. After the initial work was done, Mary's nurse kept us informed about what was happening.

"'We're not having much success,' she told us. 'We've tried just about everything. There's a weak pulse in her feet and we're using electronic devices to monitor that. There are two drugs left to try and if they don't work, there's nothing else to do.'

"One of those drugs seemed to help a little and they inserted an intra-aortic balloon up through Mary's right leg and into her heart in order to get a better blood pressure.

"Around noon on December 17, Tim Thorstonsen, a hospital chaplain, came in to see me. He was about 35, with long brown hair, and stood 6 foot 3 . He seemed to know exactly how I was feeling. Fred, Scott, and Dick had left, and I was alone and in need of human companionship.

"He [Tim] couldn't have come at a better time because shortly after we started talking, Mary's nurse came in and said that Mary was slipping and that the device in her leg was affecting the blood circulation in it.

"'What does that mean?' I asked her.

"'It means she could lose her leg,' the nurse said.

"'Then try the other one,' I said.

'She could lose that one too,' the nurse explained.

"A picture flashed through my mind of Mary without her legs. She loved to walk in the woods, cut the lawn, rush down the street to meet a friend. It was too horrible to think about, and I literally covered my face with my hands to block out that picture.

"Tim put his hand on my shoulder and said, 'There is something that might help. It's an artificial heart— called the Jarvik 7.'

"I shrugged his hand away and shook my head. Not many months before, Mary and I had watched the Barney Clark ordeal, and we decided that we'd never want anything like that done to us. We had even made out living wills asking that no artificial means be used to keep us alive. I couldn't say yes after all that.

"As we were sitting and talking, Dr. Marc Pritzger joined us. He looked sad and tired as he sat down.

"'DuWayne,' Marc said, 'we don't have any options left except the Jarvik. You've got to make a decision. I want you to call whoever you want to be here at two o'clock this afternoon to help you make it. We don't have a lot of time.'

"I called some family members and friends and we met in a big room just across the hall from Mary's room. Marc explained to all of us what her prospects were. He told us that Mary was too small for the Jarvik so a mini-Jarvik would have to be used, something that had never been tried on a human before. It would be used only as a bridge to a human heart.

"'I need to have an answer within the hour. Mary may not make it through another night,' Marc said.

"He left us then and silence descended like a shroud. I tried to open my mouth to speak but the tears started, and I couldn't get the words out. All the pressure of Mary's life was in my hands, and I couldn't forget that we had talked about these things not too long ago.

"Finally I was able to speak, and I asked if we could just go around the room and have everybody say what they thought. Their answers were always the same: 'Whatever you think is best, DuWayne.' With each answer I felt more and more alone.

"Then my good friend Curt Hedstrom said in a voice trembling with tears, 'I think we should give Mary every chance we can.'

"That helped me instantly, and I called Marc back in the room and asked if Mary was conscious. He said he thought she was, so I said I'd consent if Mary also agreed to it. He rushed across the hall to Mary's room.

"As I stepped into the hall, I suddenly realized that the whole ward, doctors, nurses, and patients were all waiting for our decision. Their eyes were fixed on Marc and Mary whom they could see from the hall. I had this weird feeling as though we were at a baseball game, and we were all facing the flag during the national anthem.

"Marc actually crawled up on the bed and was kneeling over Mary, asking her if her son's name was Scott and if her husband was DuWayne. I thought that was pretty strange at first, but then I understood he was making sure her mind was functioning normally. Then he told her she was very sick and would die without a transplant. The Jarvik heart would be used only to keep her alive until a suitable donor organ was found. He told her I had agreed, but only if she consented.

"'Do you agree, Mary?' he asked.

"'Yes,' she answered.

"With that, the whole unit gave out a yell of joy and things began to happen fast. They had already begun preparing the operating room in anticipation of our answer. Tim rushed up to tell me to come and meet Dr. Lyle Joyce, who would be doing the surgery. I had to listen to some papers read to me and then sign them. There were fourteen pages that I listened to, and I don't remember much about them until the last page which said that I consented to an autopsy in the event of Mary's death.

"I said, 'No, I can't let you do anything more to her.'

"But Mary's brother, Dick, convinced me that I should sign, and I did. The surgery began at six in the evening.

"I knew we were in for a long night, and when Tim asked us to join him for something to eat, I gladly consented. He directed us to the hospital's board room and I couldn't believe the array of food they had prepared for us. There were sandwiches, fruit, and desserts, with coffee, milk, and soft drinks. In spite of all the trauma, it tasted so good. They had also gotten rooms for us at the Wasie Building, which is attached to the hospital. I went there and showered and changed clothes while the surgery was going on.

"When I returned to the hospital, Mary Small, the director of communications came into the room where all of us were waiting and asked if she could talk with me in private. It was her job to handle the media. They were already calling for confirmation that a mini-Jarvik was being implanted in a patient. She was talking so fast that I began breathing for her, and I wanted to say 'slow down' but I didn't.

"She told me that this was a major medical event and the local and national news would soon be carrying the story. She said they wouldn't release Mary's name but only the fact that she was a 40-year-old woman from central Minnesota. She'd keep Mary's name out of the news as long as she could for the family's sake but eventually, of course, it would come out, she told me. She asked me to stay away from the media so that I wasn't recognized and bothered by them. I agreed.

"Later that evening we could see the media people, with their cameras on their shoulders, standing outside the hospital. They probably wanted a shot of Dr. Jarvik who had, just by coincidence, been at the Minneapolis/St. Paul airport at the time and he came to observe the surgery and talk to the staff. He was on his way to Washington, D.C., where hearings were going on about FDA [Food and Drug Administration] approval of the Jarvik heart.

"Surgery was finished at 12:40 A.M. One of the nurses, still dressed in scrubs, the mask hanging down around her neck, came in smiling to give us the news. Mary would be brought to the post operative care unit sometime in the early to middle morning. She suggested we all get some sleep. Scott and I went back to Wasie and got a few hours. Then we went back to the hospital. A security guard stopped us and asked who we were. I guess they were trying to keep the media out.

"Mary was in a pressurized room, and Scott and I had to scrub and dress in sterilized clothing and masks before we could go in. She wasn't awake yet, but Dr. Joyce—or Lyle as I call him—said not to worry about that because she'd been through a lot. She was on a respirator and IVs, and there was a machine about the size of a washing machine that drove the artificial heart. It went swish, swish, swish, and as I looked at my Mary lying there, I started to cry.

"Kris Johnson, Dr. Joyce's clinician, put her arms around me and said, 'It's okay. Let the tears out.' And I did.

"After I cried, Kris and I went out for a walk, and she told me that Mary had actually died for a few moments before they could get her on the bypass machine. She told me that Mary's heart had been sent away to be examined for the cause of her illness. We learned later that the heart muscle had been completely destroyed by a virus and only the Jarvik could have kept her alive. That made me feel better about my decision.

"It seemed so strange to see and hear Mary's case on every TV station and newspaper. She was making medical history, we knew, but there was something so unreal about it. Somebody from China sent us an article from a paper over there. It seemed like the whole world was waiting to see what happened to this woman from Minnesota. In a way, it made me so proud that she was brave enough to do this," DuWayne said.

Mary remained in a coma for ten days, and during that time every vital organ was affected. She was returned for surgery several times, and when her kidneys failed, she was given dialysis. She needed blood transfusions. DuWayne spent every moment that he could with her, holding her hand and talking to her. "She'd squeeze my hand and I knew she heard me," he said.

"During those long days I sat and recalled our life together. We were so much in love. I believe each of us is given one true love in life, and mine was Mary. I had met her at a harvest festival in Hoffman, Minnesota. I'd recently moved back to Minnesota from Oregon after buying 80 acres over the phone. The real-estate agent said there were woods and a duck slough, and that's all I wanted. I had just gotten out of a bad marriage and wasn't thinking about trying it again. But after meeting Mary and talking to her for five minutes (and that was about how long our first conversation was), I told my friend, 'I'm going to marry her.' She seemed so gentle and sparkly. And very pretty with auburn hair and soft hazel eyes.

"I finally got up the nerve to ask her out, and it wasn't long before we were hopelessly in love. It was a foregone conclusion that we'd get married. Mary was divorced, too, and had Scott, who was five at the time. He was like my own.

"I wanted to have a house built before we got married and I wanted to live on the land I'd bought. So we sold 40 acres of it and built the house close to the slough so we could sit and look out at the deer and rabbits and birds.

"We were married in the spring of 1975. Mary didn't like the idea of living in the country, and that was about the only problem we ever had that amounted to anything. She thought it was too dark and lonely.

"I said to her, 'I want to live here and if you don't, well, that's too bad. You'll just have to go live in the city.'

"We decided to give it a year and see how she adjusted. After that time, I asked her if she wanted to move. She said, 'If you want to go live in the city, go ahead, but I want to live here.'

"We loved going to auctions and visiting relatives for card games and homemade desserts. We had a lot of friends and family close to this area, and our lives were busy, but we always had this quiet place to come home to.

"I'd never been much of a church goer. I wasn't even confirmed. Mary was a Lutheran and went to church just about every Sunday. I decided to take confirmation instructions and join the church. I'd take a Sunday off now and then, but she wouldn't. While she was lying in that hospital bed, I'd wonder if we'd ever go and sit together as we used to and sing those slow old hymns again. Music always was a big part of her life. She loved Neil Diamond, and we'd go to his concerts when he'd come to the Cities, and it was always a big deal," DuWayne recalled.

Christmas Eve came just a few days after the Jarvik implant, and Mary was still in a coma. During the late afternoon, DuWayne walked the corridors and visited with other patients. Then he walked around the parking lot for fresh air. When he returned to their private waiting room, he couldn't believe his eyes. There in the corner was the most beautiful Christmas tree he'd ever seen, surrounded by gifts.

"There were presents for Scott and Dick and me. A bunch of postage stamps, some tee-shirts, stationery, homemade cookies, and even some wine. I said we'd save the wine for a special occasion, meaning Mary's heart transplant. It was a Christmas I'll never forget. The love and caring of that staff was incredible," he said.

On December 29 Mary awakened, moved her right arm, and wiggled her toes, an event that was broadcast across the country on the morning news. USA Today put it this way: "Mary Lund, the first woman to get an artificial heart, awoke from a coma Thursday and had to be reminded she no longer had a human heart."

A few days later, she sat on the edge of her bed and then graduated to a chair for 10 to 15 minutes. She was still on a respirator and couldn't talk, but she blinked her eyes in response to questions. When DuWayne asked her if she was afraid, she blinked yes.

Four days later she was off the ventilator and hopes were high for a human heart. Mary agreed that would be great because the artificial heart machine made so much noise it was difficult to sleep with it chugging in her ears. On January 8 her name went on the organ waiting list as a high priority and another wait began.

At 11:30 A.M. January 30, a call from Seattle ended the three-week wait. A 15-year-old girl from Billings, Montana, had had an epileptic seizure and had sustained irreversible brain damage in a fall. Tests confirmed that the heart was a match. The donor team left for Billings to retrieve the heart, and Mary cried with relief that her ordeal would soon be over. After she fell asleep, DuWayne and the other family members and staff went to their waiting room and opened that bottle of Christmas wine. "To Mary," DuWayne said as he lifted his glass. Everyone joined in that simple, elegant toast.

Mary's surgery started at 11:10 A.M. the next day, and the new heart began working immediately. DuWayne was giddy with a new-found hope that Mary's health would be restored. But by February 4, she was suffering acute shortness of breath, and she went back on the ventilator. An echocardiogram revealed that the lower portion of the heart wasn't working.

Her kidneys continued to grow weaker and her liver deteriorated. Her pancreas enlarged. Her lungs developed fibrosis. Every vital organ was affected. The ventilator and dialysis machines helped keep her alive. She was deeply depressed, as was DuWayne, and their hopes for a return to normal life were put on hold again.

Every day for the next few months, the doctors told DuWayne that Mary could die by morning. He didn't dare leave the hospital and go back home for fear something would go wrong while he was gone. He and the doctors decided together that no heroic measures would be taken to save her life.

"One day as I sat in her room talking about trivial things, I started to cry. She was still on the ventilator and couldn't talk. She touched my head with her hand and wrote on a slip of paper, 'my tough guy.' She knew I didn't cry easily," he said.

Specialists came and went, each with an expertise that seemed to be of no avail. She continued to deteriorate, and her depression escalated. In July, when things were especially bleak, DuWayne talked to her of home and things they would do together before long. Mary, agitated, pulled the oxygen mask from her face.

"Don't do that!" DuWayne said. "You could die without it."

She motioned for him to give her a pencil and paper, and she wrote "I want to see Tim." She meant Tim Thorstonsen, the hospital chaplain.

"Why?" DuWayne asked.

"He told me once that he would help me die," Mary wrote.

DuWayne knew that Tim had meant that in a spiritual sense, but Mary had taken him literally. DuWayne called Tim at home, and when Tim arrived, DuWayne left the two of them alone to talk and pray. Mary's mind was clear and reasonable, DuWayne was sure, and if she chose to die by having life support withheld, he could not disagree. She had been through more than anyone should have to endure. In spite of his love for Mary, he wouldn't encourage her to suffer more.

Tim was struck by her determination to end treatment. "We sorted that out for about an hour, both of us knowing it meant she would die very soon. I was moved by her bravery and courage just to look at that straight on, and on the other hand, moved by the incredible sense of suffering that she had endured and saw this as a release from that. It was a very poignant experience for me," Tim said.

Tim called Dr. Joyce and Dr. Pitzger and explained Mary's decision. Both doctors were resistant and reluctant to stop the process. "The staff," Tim said, "felt very connected to Mary both professionally and personally and felt there were some options that hadn't yet been tried. Both doctors met with Mary and explained that to her."

"You're getting stronger, you're tolerating food, and improving in many ways. Let's wean you off the ventilator in the next ten days," Dr. Joyce encouraged.

A psychiatrist came in to see Mary and suggested that she receive antidepressants. The medication relieved a little of the depression, but life still looked hopeless to her. By August 10, however, she was off the ventilator for a good share of the day and went for a ride with DuWayne, Dr. Joyce, and a nurse.

The next week they went out again, and this time DuWayne pushed her in a wheelchair.

They watched the ducks and geese along the water's rippled edge and recalled their own long-deserted countryside. She leaned her head against his hand and said, "Oh, DuWayne, I want to go home. I'll never complain again when I have to do the dishes, and I'll never complain when it rains. I just want to go home."

He knelt on the ground beside her and drew her into his arms. "That's all that I want, too," he whispered.

September arrived with its hint of autumn and the promise of winter in its cool evenings. DuWayne finally went home a few times to gather in the mail, which he tossed on the kitchen table, and to say hello to friends and family, whose lives had to go on. But he couldn't stay away for long. His love for Mary pulled him back to the hospital. He had no plans for the fall hunting that he had loved and no goals except to be with her every moment that he could.

Doctors and nurses began to notice that Mary was sometimes confused and disoriented and a brain scan indicated some atrophy of the brain. She became withdrawn and unresponsive. Her kidneys continued to falter, and a transplant to replace them was ruled out. By early October, she opened her eyes only when her name was spoken. Hope was fading.

It was clear to Tim Thorstonsen that it was time to speak very openly and honestly with the entire staff, who had worked for nearly a year to restore Mary's health, about her wishes to discontinue treatment.

"We gathered in the chaplain's seminar room, and every chair was taken," Tim said. "There were 23 of us. We talked about her condition and prognosis, which was very poor. I'll not forget the sense of finally coming to that consensus and people saying, 'Well, I guess that's it. It's time to stop.' It was the first time we had to face the impact of our limits and, quite frankly, our failure. It was compounded by the fact that it was a case of national interest. It was a weighty decision to end treatment, but we realized that we were no longer promoting life for Mary but only extending her dying. I tried to frame it as a gracious act of our love for Mary to let her die peacefully with some integrity.

"We took a break and someone went upstairs to get DuWayne, who was waiting for our recommendation. When he arrived, we gathered again and explained our rationale to him. All of us knew how deeply he loved Mary, and it was a painful time for us as he nodded in agreement to the inevitable."

The process was carried out very simply by withholding dialysis, and Mary slipped into a coma. Her three primary nurses had decided to all be with her and guide her through her dying. Tim was there half the time. DuWayne couldn't bear to be with her for more than a few minutes at a time. He wanted to be strong but found he couldn't.

On October 14 at 6:14 P.M., Mary died. Her struggle was finally over, but for DuWayne, a new struggle had begun.

Through the rolling, rusty autumn hills, the funeral procession carried Mary's body to the Zion Lutheran Church where friends and family, including the hospital staff, gathered for a final tribute to her extraordinary life. The strains of Mary's favorite hymn, "How Great Thou Art," reached the press, whose cameras lined the churchyard.

They carried the flower-laden casket down the steps for one final journey to the secluded cemetery where Mary would be buried. The sun glistened on the fields, and the birds dipped and dove above them. The small tent set up at the graveside couldn't hold all the guests, and Tim remembers that he walked away from it and stood looking over the fields instead of at the grave, watching the birds in what seemed to be a celebration dance of freedom.

After the funeral guests had left, DuWayne was alone in the house where he and Mary had lived for 10 years. Every corner of it spoke of her: the antiques they had collected and refinished, the ceramic dishes she had painted with such care, and the blouse that hung on the closet door just as she had left it.

In the kitchen, nearly a year's worth of mail was strewn carelessly on the table and counter. DuWayne shoved it aside and sat down. During the months of her illness, he had been able to push away his own despair in order to give her hope. Now there was no need of that. He sat looking at his hands, turning over in his mind a thought that kept recurring since her death. He didn't want to live without her.

"I thought of the days and years ahead of me, and I couldn't stand it. I wanted to die, too. I thought about how I would end my life—a shot to the brain, carbon monoxide poison, sleeping pills.

"But then I started thinking about the church's teaching. I was taught that if you took your own life, you couldn't enter heaven, and then I'd never see Mary again. I decided that night that I'd have to live out my life to its natural end in order to be with her."

And so he began his journey back to life. It began by crying—finally letting out the well of tears that he had so seldom shed.

"I cried and cried. I just couldn't stop. Some little thing would remind me of her, and the tears would come without warning," he recalled.

"I tried to go back to church, but I would start to cry after a few minutes and I'd get up and leave. Now I don't go anymore. I'm not mad at the church and I'm not mad at God, but I can't be in that building. We sat there side by side through many Sunday mornings, and then she was buried from that church. I guess the memories are just too painful for me."

DuWayne has chosen to stay in their home, going to work at night to avoid the evenings alone. His close circle of friends, including some of the hospital staff, has been his salvation. He lives day to day, without too many plans or goals. His one wish is that he could dream of Mary, but he can't.

"That's the only way I can see her moving and talking," he said. But with one exception shortly after her death, his wish has eluded him.

He keeps in touch with Mary's donor family, exchanging Christmas cards each year.

"It isn't that we want to become friends or get better acquainted. We just want to communicate once in a while. The donor's parents contacted me after Mary died to tell me how sorry they were. It might have seemed that their daughter died twice. I don't know. It would have been so great for them if Mary had lived," he said.

He's grateful for the years they shared together, and he feels the same depth of pride today as he did when Mary first agreed to participate in an experiment that would advance medical knowledge.

"She's part of history now," he said. "I thought of that when I chose the inscription on her tombstone. I wanted people to know a hundred or two hundred years from now what she had done."

In the small, secluded cemetery, he has placed a monument that will last at least that long.

It reads:

> On December 18, 1985 Mary Lund became the first woman ever to receive a total artificial heart. On Jan. 31, 1986 she was transplanted with a human heart. She lived courageously, enriched all our lives, and greatly enhanced medical knowledge, ensuring the life of future transplant recipients. I loved her very much.

Guidepost: The Most Difficult Decision

The suddenness of Mary's illness left Mary and DuWayne unprepared for the ordeal they had to face. Yet their extraordinary courage captured the attention of people around the world. They had taken every step possible to save Mary's life. Yet, medical science couldn't undo the damage her illness had waged.

And when it was time to make the decision to let Mary go, the entire family of health care providers that made up Mary's team helped DuWayne accept Mary's final wish: respite from her lengthy and exhausting illness.

In the face of such crises, decision making will always be difficult and sometimes impossible for those most involved. The support of clergy, psychologists, social workers, hospital staff, family, and friends is essential. Yet, the decisions made by those who love the patient should never be allowed to overrule the ultimate authority the patient must be allowed to have over his or her own destiny.

DuWayne's love for Mary allowed her that dignity.

7

Cal: Charting a New Course

Cal Stoll became famous as a coach for the Minnesota Gophers football team from 1972 to 1978. Now he's famous as an evangelist, preaching the good news of organ transplantation and the legacy of organ donation. He travels from coast to coast, always giving credit to his hero—the man whose heart is now his own.

Cal received his new heart on July 23, 1987. This former cigar-smoking coach, along with three other heart recipients, founded the Second Chance for Life Foundation in 1989 to pass along this gift of life. He talks to groups of any size, in any place, to tell them about this new treatment, which can take place only when grief-stricken families offer life through organ donations.

Cal knows what death looks like. The doctors at the University of Minnesota Hospitals had given him 24 hours to live, and 18 of those hours had ticked away before someone somewhere offered the organs of a family member who had suffered brain death. The heart was the size and blood type that Cal needed. At the age of 63, he exchanged death for life.

The story of his medical problems began 13 years before. Cal decided that when he turned 50 he should have a thorough medical check-up, so he made an appointment at the Mayo Clinic. They put him through the paces, including a stress test. After looking at the results, a doctor asked, "When did you have your heart attack?"

"I never had one," Cal answered.

"Oh yes you did. You've got to start taking better care of yourself," the doctor told him. "Stop smoking, get in shape, lose some weight."

When he left the hospital, Cal threw his last two cigars across the parking lot and hasn't had one since. He began dieting and exercising and lost 20 pounds. Coaching was his life, and he kept up a busy pace, occasionally feeling some discomfort but ignoring it.

After a year he went back for another check-up. This time, they wouldn't put him on the stress machine at all.

"You've had another heart attack in the last ten days," the doctor said.

"No I haven't," Cal replied.

"Yes, you have. Take it easy for six weeks and come back for another check-up," the doctor said.

During those six weeks, Cal suffered chest pains regularly and ate nitroglycerin like it was popcorn. But when he went back for an angiogram, it showed there was nothing wrong with his heart. He dumped out his nitroglycerin and went home.

For ten years, Cal led a normal life, coaching and traveling. Then in 1985 he began to show symptoms of heart failure. He had shortness of breath, retention of fluids, and loss of energy.

"I was back on medication and doing all right," Cal said. "In 1986 I went to coach an Italian football team for seven months. My wife, June, was with me. After we left Italy, we spent some time in Paris and Copenhagen, and in London I really started to feel the effects of heart failure. By the time we got home in August, I was going down hill rapidly. By December, I couldn't comb my hair or brush my teeth.

"I sat up all night with my head on my chest, trying to breathe because every time I'd lie down I'd start to drown in my own fluids. I went to one cardiologist, and I decided he was trying to kill me so I quit seeing him.

"Then I went to the University of Minnesota where I should have gone in the first place. After a check-up by Dr. Jay Cohen, he asked me, 'What about a heart transplant?'

"I unbuttoned my shirt and said, 'Let's go in the morning.' I knew I was older than most transplants, but they were willing to consider me. They put me through the work-up, and I was accepted on the list. I guess waiting to know whether or not I could get on the list was the only trauma I've had. I've never had any misgivings, no mood swings, no depression. I'm the luckiest guy in the world."

Cal waited for six and a half months to become that lucky guy.

"I never thought about dying," he said. "I refused to. I think you can will yourself to die or not to die, and unless a superior being made that decision for me, I wasn't going to die."

Cal spent the first months of waiting at home with a beeper beside him. One night he was awakened by a "beep, beep, beep," and he nudged his wife and said, "Honey, let's go get my new heart." But when he reached for the beeper, he realized the sound wasn't coming from it. It was the smoke alarm in the hall. The batteries were getting low and it was sending out its warning.

The next time he heard the beeper go off, he waited for a while. Then he called the transplant office and said, "Have you got my heart?"

"No, we didn't call you. Check the batteries on your beeper."

Sure enough, they were getting low, too.

By early June his condition had deteriorated further and he was admitted to the hospital. He went from 225 to 150 pounds, clinging to life one hour at a time. On July 22, the doctors came in and said, "Coach, if something drastic doesn't happen in the next 24 hours, we can't make any promises."

"Just go find the heart," Cal whispered. "I'll do the rest."

And on July 23, 1987, a night most Twin Cities residents remember as the night of the hundred-year flood, Cal got his heart.

As he puts it, "There was thunder and lightning, the rains came down, the Lord spoke, and Cal got his new heart." And, as he promised, he did the rest.

Within 13 days he was out of the hospital. Within the month, he was driving a car and going to work. And he's a happy, happy man despite his new lifestyle.

"My toenails fall out. My ankles swell. I've had shingles and energy swings. I grow hair in funny places and grow fat where I shouldn't. My balance is affected and I fall down once in a while. I have no feeling on the top of my feet, but I don't worry about it because they still work. I had a chance to avoid all these problems by dying, so I never complain."

"And, by the way, there is sex after transplantation. I know there are cases of impotence among transplants. Medication might accelerate it, as well as fear. I asked my 90-year-old grandfather how old I have to be to stop worrying about sex. He said, 'You'll have to ask somebody older than me.'

"I have my own principles of longevity. First is attitude—putting everything in the proper perspective, changing what you can and not worrying about the things you can't. Second is understanding your medication. Know the side-effects. Listen to your body. Let it talk to you. Third, eat right and exercise. That's all there is to it.

"The sooner you take control of your life after transplantation, the better chance you have of a quality life. But if you lie around and feel sorry for yourself, you're in trouble. You don't get something for nothing in this world. We traded death for a lifetime of medical management. Living with an attitude of compliance, I'll live forever."

Cal likes to quote William James, who said, "The greatest use of life is to spend it on something that outlives it."

And Cal tries to do that. In six months, he gave more than 200 talks about the wonders of transplantation and the need for more donors. "Someone had to die so I could live. On the day he died, he left the greatest legacy that any one human being could leave another—the gift of life—and he's my hero.

"If we could get everybody in this country educated in the next 20 years about donating organs, we wouldn't have a problem of short supply," he said.

Cal sees a need to have people trained throughout the country to work with donor families. The counselors must be people who understand the total concept, understand what has to happen and the chronology of what happens, and who possess a deep compassion for people going through the trauma of a sudden death. And that shouldn't be

Transplants: Unwrapping the Second Gift of Life

someone who's been in the operating room for hours trying to save that life.

He hopes that someday a monument to donors will be constructed as a visible symbol of appreciation to them and their heroic families.

He keeps in touch with many donor families and with all the heart transplants from the University of Minnesota. He can rattle off the names of each, the dates of their surgery, and how they're doing. His meticulous notebook includes addresses and phone numbers and for some, the date and cause of death. Those are sad entries for Cal to make because he sees every recipient as a member of his extended family.

Those activities are all goals of the Second Chance nonprofit, volunteer organization of which he's president. Its long-range goals include establishing a National Heart Day to educate and encourage organ donation and to demonstrate to the community the success of transplantation and the quality of life it allows. Second Chance also hopes to set up a fund to assist in paying for medication and other related costs for those in need, and to publish a low-sodium, low-cholesterol, low-calorie cook book.

Cal and June live in a large, comfortable home that reflects June's design and art background. Cal works at home editing the *Second Chance Newsletter* and keeping a calendar of speaking engagements. June is his quiet support, traveling with him to out-of-state appointments.

"We have the same mental attitudes," she said. "After 41 years, you kind of blend. And Cal really hasn't changed at all. He never complains and I really haven't had to make any adjustments."

Perhaps he hasn't changed much. He used to play football with everything he had. Now he preaches the good news of heart transplantation with the same dedication and enthusiasm. The crowds that applaud him are a little smaller now but the cause is bigger than winning a game.

Guidepost: Quality of Life

Cal Stoll is a transplant program's dream. Although he was past the average age for such a procedure, doctors found he possessed the criteria they were looking for.

First, Cal's mental attitude was positive. He didn't spend time debating whether or not he should have the transplant. He knew immediately that he couldn't pass up the opportunity to live a healthy life again.

He willingly complies with the medical regimen and works hard to maintain an appropriate diet and exercise routine; he keeps scheduled doctor appointments. His new lifestyle, while not without difficulties, is a constant source of joy for him.

He carries that joy wherever he goes, and people he meets find it contagious. That's perhaps his greatest gift to prospective or new transplant recipients. He serves as a role model who exemplifies the new quality of life an organ recipient can attain.

Many of the people I've interviewed are making similar contributions, each in his or her own way. While it's certainly not a requirement, I can tell you those who reach out to others, when they're ready to do so, seem to find a special fulfillment that adds to their quality of life.

Transplants: Unwrapping the Second Gift of Life

8

Larry: Sailing for Strength

When Larry Atkin goes sailing this summer, it won't be an ordinary day. It will be another milestone in his incredible journey back to life. His restored Chris Craft boat, the Champlain, will carry young cancer patients, and Larry hopes the boat will inspire them as it did him in his struggle against pancreatic cancer.

His cancer was diagnosed in April, 1988, and his prognosis was grave. "Larry, you have only four to six weeks to live," doctors told him.

"For a week, my family and I cried," Larry remembered. "I took walks in the park near our house and felt a closeness to nature I had never felt before. How short our lives really are. I saw older people and I envied them. I loved them for reaching old age and I wanted to grow old, too.

"That was a hard week, but I decided to fight back. I talked to doctors, healers, yogis, psychologists, dietitians and friends, and then I remembered my old model Chris Craft. My grandfather Nathan had given it to me on my fifteenth birthday in 1957. I'd been looking at it in the store window for a long time. I was so happy when I unwrapped that package and I put the boat together in my parents' basement woodshop. Then I set it on a shelf and it stayed there for 32 years," he said.

But, during those traumatic days of discovering his life was ending, Larry began to remember his childhood, his parents, his boyhood friends. "I needed to be in touch with 'the good old days,' and I retrieved my model Chris Craft, wiped off the dust, and decided to refinish her, giving her a new coat of paint and revarnishing her decks and cabin. On one of those evenings as I sat working on her, I daydreamed about sailing the 'real thing' and a feeling of *deja vu* came over me. I remembered being 15 and daydreaming that same dream of sailing the 'real thing.' What a challenge to find and restore a real cruiser and restore my life at the same time. To beat this thing called cancer!

"I knew I had only a three percent chance of survival after five years. It would be a further challenge to restore a classic Chris Craft cabin cruiser at the same time. I started my search for a boat about 40 feet long, from the early 1950's, one that would hold my family for those long cruises down the East Coast, and around Lake Champlain in Vermont, where we live," he said.

"In June of 1988, in a small town about 15 miles from my home, I noticed several large boats in dry dock under winter covers. One drew me closer. I peeked under the blue cover and it didn't take me long to realize that this was the very same boat that I had built in model form those many years ago—and it was for sale. The cancer had met its match. If I could resurrect this hulk with its massive areas of rotting wood, then I could master my own body," Larry said.

But it was not to be. When Larry called the owner, he discovered the cost was exorbitant and, deeply disappointed, Larry told the owner he couldn't afford it.

Then, toward the end of July, Larry, his wife, Christina, and sons, William and Lee, took a cruise on the St. Lawrence River. Near Quebec City, they saw a sister ship to the one he couldn't afford back home. "She was gleaming in the distance and beckoned me aboard," Larry said. "I resolved to plead with the owner to reduce the price. My life was at stake here."

After some hard negotiations, Larry bought the boat that August. "She was called 'Champlain' and was a 1951 Chris Craft, 42 foot, double-cabin, flying-bridge cruiser. She was an original and she was dying. Her engines were dead, her bowels wrought with holes," he recalled.

But the Champlain went through a transformation, as did Larry. He threw himself into the restoration almost as if the mending of the boat and his own healing were intertwined. When his chemotherapy made him sick and he couldn't sleep, he'd work on the boat. When he wasn't well enough to work, he'd lie in bed, planning the next phase of repair. He was in a race and there were going to be two winners.

But Larry's chemotherapy had no beneficial effect, and his new diet wasn't making much difference either. The boat work became more and more important to him because it provided the will to go on. Sometimes, after a chemo treatment, he could hardly climb the ladder to the cabin, but through sheer force of will, he dragged himself up.

"I knew I needed some drastic medical attention. My physical condition was getting in the way of my boat building and I couldn't allow that. Then, through a family member, I met an attorney from Hartford, Connecticut, with the same condition I had. He had had a liver transplant as well as pancreatic surgery. He was playing tennis now. He was well!" Larry said.

Larry was determined to explore the transplant option. At Hartford Hospital, he met with Dr. Robert Schweitzer, a transplant surgeon who suggested he undergo the myriad tests in preparation for being placed on the list to receive a liver transplant. Once the okay was given, he waited for three agonizing weeks before a suitable donor was found.

"I had to be ready to fly to Connecticut at a moment's notice and be prepared for surgery that could last up to 28 hours and a stay in the hospital of up to six weeks. I wouldn't be able to work for an additional 25 weeks, not an easy thought for a self-employed architect," Larry recalled.

"Finally, on Valentine's Day, 1990, I flew to Hartford to have my transplant and Whipple procedure (the removal of most of my pancreas, the lower one-third of my stomach, my duodenum, gall bladder, and some other assorted parts). The surgery lasted 13 hours, with three surgeons participating. Doctors called it a textbook operation—each maneuver went easily.

"I recuperated in the hospital for six weeks, thinking and planning my work on the boat. And in the process, I built another even larger boat model. It was so large that the doctors gave me the hospital room reserved for the Governor and other dignitaries. The room was huge and had a great view. The doctors told me I could go home after I finished the model, and when I was done, I was really ready to go home," Larry laughed.

But Larry found that his muscles had been weakened during his hospitalization and he could barely walk. Slowly he began exercising on a trampoline and his body responded. He regained his strength and his normal weight and soon he was once again climbing the ladder to the boat that had served as a symbol of hope through his long journey.

He has had virtually no side effects from the liver transplant, but the Whipple surgery is another matter. "I'm able to separate the two procedures," Larry said. "I haven't had any liver rejection and I've never been hospitalized since my surgery, but my digestive process is what causes me the most trouble because so much of my intestines are gone. I have to be very careful about what I eat."

Larry doesn't complain about much. He's too happy to be alive and sailing the Champlain. And to share his renewed life, he's joined an American Cancer Society volunteer group and offers cruises to young cancer patients and their families.

"The Champlain has the capacity to transform the lives of others as she did mine," Larry said wistfully. "I'm looking forward to lots of happy sailing."

Guidepost: Mobilizing Your Passion

Larry's passion for that classic Chris Craft, like Cal Stoll's positive attitude, contributed to his healing. Focusing on something that required all of his attention and provided him the positive rewards he had dreamed about for years undoubtedly set him back on a path toward life. His "overcomer's" attitude indeed helped him to beat that cancer.

Mobilizing our passions—finding something that interests us to distraction and requires us to dig deep down into our creative selves—is surely an important part of healing. Larry's strong desire to realize his dream brought him back to life in attitude and gave him the will to overcome illness. Today his work is bringing enjoyment to cancer patients and their families, inspiring them to discover their own creative passions.

9

Ardelle: Hints of Trouble on the Road Ahead

I clutched the arm of my airline seat. I hate flying and in October 1990, as we approached the San Francisco airport, it looked as if we'd land in the middle of San Francisco Bay. I sighed with relief as I felt the reassuring thud of wheels on solid ground.

I was on my way to California to be with Ardelle for her check-up at Stanford, something she had been putting off for far too long. It had been over a year since her last heart biopsy and the entire family was concerned.

After her check-up, she would join me in Dallas to visit Dr. Maria Teresa Olivari, who had been part of the University of Minnesota team when Ardelle had her transplant. I chose to visit the Southwestern University transplant program because I knew Dr. Olivari (or Mother Teresa as she's called by those who have been under her loving care) would have an outstanding program.

I scanned the crowded airport terminal until I found Ardelle and her son-in-law, Solie. She had told me on the phone that she had lost a lot of weight since I had last seen her, and indeed she had. She looked trim and tanned.

Except for the pain in her hips, which made walking difficult, she seemed in good spirits and health.

We checked into our motel, and in the morning we went to her appointment with Dr. Shirley Hunt of the Stanford Heart Transplant Program.

After checking her vital signs, Dr. Hunt scheduled Ardelle for blood tests and x-rays that afternoon, and a biopsy and angiogram the next morning.

As we left the hospital by taxi, we had our first real look at the beautiful Stanford campus. The red-tiled roofs, the green expanses of lawn with their stately palms, and the clear blue sky created an indelible picture of California beauty.

Later, Ardelle and I settled into bed, each with our own books and our own thoughts. I felt her unspoken dread of the next day's tests even after the lights were out and the hum of California traffic filled the room.

By 6:30 A.M., we were on our way back to the hospital. The biopsy Ardelle had dreaded went off without a hitch. When the procedure is done with skilled hands, it can be quick and relatively painless. But after some bad experiences with clumsy interns, Ardelle had developed a quite rational fear of biopsies.

When I went to see her in the recovery room, she was sleepy and relieved that it was over. The doctors wouldn't allow her to fly with me to Dallas so soon after the procedure, so I had to leave without her, though she would join me the next day. Before I left for the airport, I pinched her toe and said good-bye.

I arrived in Dallas about eleven at night and couldn't find a shuttle. After waiting for an hour, I was about ready to call a taxi even though I had learned that the fare would be $23. As I was sitting on my suitcase pondering this, a taxi drove up. The driver asked where I wanted to go and how much the shuttle would cost. "Ten dollars," I told him.

"I'm just calling it quits for the night and I want to make some money on the way home. I'll take you for the same price as the shuttle," he said. "That's a deal," I told him, and sank into the back seat. Traveling in a strange city, even in the best of health, can be a trial, I discovered.

It was midnight by the time I got settled in the hotel but in California it was only ten o'clock so I called to see if Ardelle had gotten back to her room and if she had any results from her tests.

When I reached her, I found the news wasn't good. The echocardiogram indicated that something was wrong. Dr. Hunt had told her it was either rejection or the amyloid attacking her new heart as it had done the original. We knew the amyloidosis was still in her body, but we hadn't counted on this.

"Dr. Hunt said she'll have the conclusive reports back tomorrow," Ardelle said.

"Have you called the twins?" I asked.

"No. It's too late, and besides we really don't have much to tell them yet," Ardelle said.

"I'll be at the airport to meet you tomorrow," I told her. "Try to get some sleep and I'll see you then."

I felt the bottom had fallen out of everything. We were back to square one, it seemed. In the morning I called

Marilyn to tell her our news and just to hear her voice. I felt so alone and hopeless. I knew Ardelle felt the same—and worse.

Late in the afternoon I went to the airport to meet Ardelle. We took the shuttle back to the hotel and decided to go out for dinner. Over a glass of wine, we laughed and talked as we always had, but I was thinking, "Here we are, two sisters growing older, visiting a city we'll probably never visit together again." I wanted to cry, but I kept on laughing.

In the morning we went to the hospital to meet Dr. Olivari. When she saw Ardelle, she threw her arms around her.

"You look wonderful!" the doctor exclaimed. "You've lost a lot of weight!"

"I've still got a little tummy, though," Ardelle said.

"Come into the office and tell me about the tests. Do you have any reports with you?" the doctor asked.

"No, I have to call Dr. Hunt at Stanford later today to find out specifically what they show," Ardelle told her.

"Well, you know if it's the amyloid attacking the heart, there's nothing that can be done. Certain kinds of rejection can be treated. Others can't," she explained.

"Dr. Hunt will send all the reports to you, to the University of Minnesota, and to my doctor in Ukiah so everybody will know what's happening," Ardelle said.

We stayed only a short time. Now we had a long day ahead of us, including a three-hour tour of Dallas.

When the tour was over, we went to our hotel to call Dr. Hunt for the report on Ardelle's heart. I watched Ardelle's face as she listened to the doctor. I saw her eyes fill with tears and when she hung up, she said, "It's the amyloid. There's nothing that can be done."

We shed many tears as we called our sisters and Ardelle's daughter, Julie. Jon, her son, had left on a hunting trip that morning so we couldn't reach him.

Because Ardelle was only the second person in the world to receive a heart transplant after having her own heart attacked by amyloidosis, there was virtually no data on life expectancy. She had just been given a death sentence with an undetermined stay of execution. Ardelle's acceptance of the news amazed me.

"I'm more concerned about how this will affect my kids and my three sisters, than myself," she told me.

"Would you go through another transplant if it was offered?" I asked her.

"No," she answered, "and it would never be offered. The amyloid would probably attack that one, too. Besides, I think I'm still in shock from the first one," she quipped. "You know I'd never been sick in my entire life until that happened, and I'd never been in the hospital except when I had the kids."

"Do you ever regret having it?" I asked.

She hesitated: "Well, no, I guess not. I saw a new grandchild I wouldn't have seen, and I've watched the others grow a little older."

"Did you feel at all that the family pushed you too hard to have it?" That had been a concern of ours because Ardelle had been reluctant at first and we had urged her to accept another chance at life.

"I told Dr. Herzog at Hennepin County Hospital that I

didn't dare say no after everything the family and the doctors had done to get me on the list. I didn't want anybody to be mad. I guess I just went along with the tide," she said.

"What has been the biggest problem for you?" I asked.

"I hated the way I looked. It was terrible, just terrible. And then when I went back to Alaska and no one recognized me I felt like a ghost. People would look right at me and not know me. I didn't want to go out and have people see me," she recalled.

"Living with Marilyn and Peter that first year after the transplant was really good, though. Marilyn just let me take over the kitchen and do whatever I wanted. When Peter came home, we'd sit and watch a little TV together and talk. Then I'd make dinner so when Marilyn came home from work she wouldn't have to cook. Marion came from Phoenix and stayed a whole month, too, you know. I was well taken care of.

"But Alaska was weird. After I started losing weight I began to look more like myself, and then it wasn't so bad. The newspaper up there did a story on me, and one day I was walking down the mall and there I was, on the front page of the paper. I was really shocked. I hadn't expected front-page coverage!

"You know," she said, "another thing that really bothers me is the fragile skin. I just barely touch something and it rips. At Marilyn's I tore it on the cupboard, at Julie's on the closet door, and at Jon's on the shower door, so I've got scars from everywhere I've gone. Then last week I ripped my arm at the laundromat.

"Sometimes, at the most unlikely times, I remember I have another person's heart in me, and that gives me a funny feeling. But I don't think I was ever depressed. Otherwise, I think I've done pretty well. But there are so many things I can't do anymore. I used to be in such good shape, but this has really aged me. The osteoporosis bothers me a lot. It hurts to bend over even to make a bed.

"And now, after everything we've all been through, the amyloid is back. Those little monsters! Those little heart-eaters!" she exclaimed.

I laughed at her characterization, which made me envision small Pac Men nibbling at her heart.

"Okay, let's get serious again," I said. "Are there things you want to live for, some goals you've set?"

"Not really. Yes, there was one. I always wanted to write a book—a romance. I could see it in my mind, but I never got started," she sighed.

I recalled she had mentioned this to me in the past, but I didn't realize until that moment it had been an unfulfilled lifetime dream. I felt sad and somehow guilty that I was fulfulling my writing dream because of her experience with a transplant, while she again faced the deadly mysterious disease that was destroying her life.

We tried to recapture the joy of being together, but both of us were slipping into longer and longer silences, watching meaningless television. I wanted nothing more than to go home to my daughter Clair, my friend Kasey, and my warm, comforting cats. Getting such news in a hotel room far from home was something we hadn't expected and were ill prepared for. Ardelle took the lead in shaking us out of our depression.

"Come on," she said. "We've got an evening and a day left together so let's get dressed up and go out for dinner."

I pressed my wrinkled clothes and put on lipstick. I thought, "If she can be brave, I guess I'd better try, too." We went to our hotel restaurant and ordered a glass of wine and a light dinner and spent the evening making silly toasts to each other and reminiscing. It was difficult for me to gauge what was going on inside my sister's mind. She seemed unbelievably gracious in accepting her fate. I felt if I were in her place, I would be railing against it with all my might. Still, I had not lived her life or thought her thoughts, so it was impossible for me to judge her reaction.

The Dallas morning was cool and bright when we awoke. Ardelle wanted to get some presents for her grandchildren so we took off to do some shopping. We had been told there was very little shopping in downtown Dallas so we asked our taxi driver to take us to a shopping area outside of town that we had found in the Yellow Pages. We had no idea where it was, and he didn't seem to either.

Ardelle and I formed a mini-friendship with the cab driver on the way to our destination. He told us about his son, who at age 15 had died for lack of a heart transplant, and he told us how brave his son had been.

"I guess if he could go through all that stuff without any fear I can face life without fear, too, and with kindness toward other people." I thought how very much alike his son and my sister were.

When we finally arrived, the driver said, "I'd better wait for you. You'll never get a cab to come all the way out here. I'll give you a special deal on the fare if you want me to wait." I agreed.

The shopping area we found held a series of stalls full of jewelry, clothing, toys, and gadgets. Ardelle was an ardent shopper in spite of her painful hips, and we found the presents she needed. When we were done, the driver was waiting for us, and we went back to the hotel with our treasures.

We awoke early the next morning despite our late night, and we packed our suitcases, stuffing our presents between layers of clothing. The trip to the Dallas/Ft. Worth Airport was our last ride together. Ardelle was heading back to San Francisco and I to Minneapolis. Our gates were separated by a long walk, so we said our farewell at hers. We held each other for a long time, both of us in tears. But as usual, she was the brave one.

"Now don't cry, Pat. You go home and write your book and don't worry about anything else," she whispered.

I left her there and walked toward my gate. I didn't turn around and wave. I just kept walking, looking for my gate through a kaleidoscope of tears.

Transplants: Unwrapping the Second Gift of Life

10

Kelly, Crosby, and Mary: Travel Guides

As I began to learn more about organ transplantation, I made a point of meeting and spending time with people who could help me understand how transplants change lives.

One of these helpful guides is Kelly Prindle, a transplant social worker in Dallas. Kelly and I talked about many aspects of transplantation and life afterwards. Her job is to evaluate the psychosocial health of the prospective recipient and the recipient's family. She offers supportive counseling throughout the process of assessment, transplant, and post-transplant experiences.

She had just returned from the annual conference of heart transplant social workers and had updated information on the issues that are of most concern to recipients. One study centered on the incidence and frequency of medication side-effects and the stress level associated with each. Since the medications can't be stopped because of the certainty of rejection, their side-effects must be dealt with and monitored.

"Changed body appearance was a top one, especially for women," she said. "The weight gain, the round face, the hair growth, the fat deposits on the back and stomach contribute to feelings of insecurity about one's appearance. Marital difficulties may result because of faulty conclusions such as

'My mate doesn't think I'm attractive anymore.' Increased hair growth on the face and back is a real problem for women. We don't encourage electrolysis or waxing because they can cause infection or irritation. Most women use a depilatory and a few shave their arms because of the excess hair."

Altered vision, whether better or worse, may occur due to the different medications taken post-transplant. Some patients complain of watery eyes.

"Our program suggests recipients wait for at least six months before changing their eye prescriptions since the alteration might take that long to stabilize," she explained.

Depression was another concern. Transplantation is emotionally draining. The initial feelings of euphoria at having a second chance at life eventually taper to a time of emotional adjustment, including depression, mood swings, and even temporary psychosis. Many people mistakenly interpret a recipient's depression as a lack of gratitude toward the family or the transplant. In some instances, depression is the physical response of the body to high doses of new medication.

Patients are concerned about sexual issues, too. "Our transplant manual simply states, 'Sexual activity is not prohibited.' However, the coordinators review this information with the patient and family during the post-transplant teaching and encourage questions. Many patients have concerns about sexual problems, but they are afraid to ask. Sexual dysfunction occurs frequently," Kelly said.

Some common reasons for sexual dysfunction in the transplant patient are recovery from surgery, fear of a heart attack, fear of dysfunction, fear of harming oneself, low self-esteem, body image concerns, family conflict, and depression.

Medication can affect sexual desire, too. Some medications result in fatigue, yeast infections in women, outbreaks of herpes, and genital warts. High blood pressure medication can cause impotence in males, decreased libido, and decreased lubrication in women. Steroid-induced diabetes can decrease sexual functioning and desire.

Some couples have marital problems that revolve around the sexual issue. Frequently, unresolved marital problems exist in a marriage before transplant. The couples will go to great lengths to get the patient to transplant, and when the immediate threat of death has passed, the unresolved issues resurface. Kelly refers patients and their families to a private counselor if she believes marital counseling is required.

Tremors, or the "cyclosporine shakes" affect many people, too. This slight trembling is noticeable mostly in the hands and can be a nuisance while eating or drinking or doing detailed work.

Some recipients complain about a lack of sleep because of the need to urinate frequently. Weight gain—often blamed on steroids, which can increase appetite—is a constant source of frustration for many. Fragile skin is another complaint since it can be unsightly and conducive to infection.

"Just hitting your arm or hand on a belt buckle, for instance, can tear the skin," Kelly said.

I told her that Ardelle's arms and legs were full of little bruises and cuts, and because her immune system is suppressed by the drugs, Ardelle is always concerned about infection. Many people, including Ardelle, suffer from swollen ankles, headaches, and bone deterioration.

"When post-transplant people talk to those contemplating transplant, I encourage them to discuss both pros and cons so people can make informed decisions. Sometimes the post-transplant people paint a one-sided picture and never tell the patient about the potential disadvantages," Kelly said.

The one-year anniversary seems to be a big milestone for transplant patients. "There's a new sense of self-confidence that they've survived the first year and things are going to get even better," said Kelly. "But life will never be like it was, and people find a new normal in their lives. We don't want people to have unrealistic expectations about life after transplantation. You're exchanging one set of problems that you know will lead to death for the opportunity to live again with a whole new set of potential problems.

"One of the most distressing problems after transplant," Kelly went on, "is the continued uncertainty of rejection and infection. Recipients often worry about time off from work because of doctor's visits or unforeseen complications. When recipients return to work and stop receiving disability payments, many still feel emotionally disabled and unequipped for the stress of work. The transplant team then faces a dilemma because, from a cardiac standpoint, the recipient is physically capable of returning to work and can't be considered disabled."

Not surprisingly, recipients are curious about their donors. "In our program, we keep all donor information confidential to protect both the donor family and the recipient,"

Kelly said. This is done to avoid any feelings of ownership on the part of the donor family and feelings of obligation on the part of the recipient. Some recipients have a difficult time expressing their gratitude because "thank you" doesn't seem adequate. However, most recipients do want to write an anonymous letter of thanks to the donor family, and some send a note every year on their transplant anniversary.

The organ procurement agency receives the letters and contacts the donor family to see if they wish to receive any correspondence from the recipient. The organ procurement agency reserves the right to screen letters for appropriateness and anonymity.

With heart transplants, social workers discuss the myths of the heart with the patient before transplant. One of these myths is that the patient's personality will change as a result of receiving another person's heart. There is sometimes the fear that if a man gets a woman's heart he may become feminine or may not be interested in hobbies he once enjoyed.

"There is much mystery woven around the heart, and it's hard to put aside in a matter of weeks what's been fabricated for years," Kelly said.

In the middle of our conversation, we suddenly heard a woman's voice call out, "Oh God, oh no!" followed by deep sobs. Kelly rushed to the next office to see what had happened. I could hear her say, "I know you worked so hard to keep him alive." The sobs continued.

When Kelly came back, she told me that someone waiting for a heart had died. Kelly's co-worker, who had spent a great deal of time with the patient in rehabilitation, had just learned of the patient's death and was grief-stricken. I saw firsthand the toll this life and death drama takes on hospital staff.

Soon Crosby Uwagbai, a student from Nigeria, arrived at Kelly's office, his arms laden with art work he had done. After introducing ourselves, I looked through his drawings of faces and masks. He explained that many of his drawings and sculptures were going to be auctioned off to raise funds for people who needed transplants and post-transplant medication.

"Why are you doing this?" I asked.

"Because I want to give something back to the people and the hospital who have helped me live. I want other people to be able to live, too," he told me.

Crosby came to Dallas from Nigeria in 1981 to study, but he also needed to work and got a job as a security guard.

"I was always walking outside and I got a bad cold and was sick for about eight months," Crosby said. "The doctor gave me medicine, but it didn't work, so I went back to see him again because my feet were swollen. They gave me all kinds of medication, but nothing helped. Then I met Dr. Yancey, who saw my problem and said I needed a heart transplant.

"I was lucky that I only waited three weeks for a donor and then I was transplanted on February 4, 1990. I stayed in the hospital one week. I feel good. I feel great. I have so much energy today," he said.

The biggest hurdle for Crosby is taking the medication and knowing he'll be doing that for the rest of his life.

"You have to learn to manage your time so you can take your medication, and you have to learn to live with little aches and pains. But that's all better than dying. I've got a puffy face and I'm always hungry, but I've tried to cut down what I eat.

"Every day I wake up and feel good. I'm surprised I'm here, and I say, 'thank God.' Your perspective on life changes. My property, such as clothes, doesn't matter anymore. It's people who matter.

"When I got sick, I didn't have insurance or anything. People helped me to get Medicaid funds to pay for the transplant. And when I got well, I said, 'I'm going to do something in return.' That's why I'm giving my art to be sold for the transplant program."

Crosby's wife, Elizabeth, is also a student, and they have two sons.

"I have a wonderful wife," Crosby said. "Not all wives could be so patient with a husband, but she was always there. And she's still here now, and my two boys are here, too. In the morning, I look into their eyes and I think, 'I have to keep on going.' They are my reason to live, and I don't have time to be depressed. The love you share with your family and friends makes you want to live."

Crosby praised the Southwestern/St.Paul Medical Center staff and said that if he's feeling bad and comes to the hospital, he starts feeling better as soon as he gets to the door.

"They make me feel at home because they talk to me and they really care about me. They want me to be here," Crosby said.

He's had some inflammation of the gums because of the cyclosporine, and the doctors have cautioned him not to lift anything too heavy. Other than that, Crosby feels that his life is getting back to normal in less than a year after transplant.

He takes good care of himself and never misses an appointment with the doctor, accepting the biopsies as something he has to do to maintain his health. He tries not to nap in the afternoon and to drink less water in the evening so his night's sleep isn't interrupted too much by trips to the bathroom.

He explained that the doctors told him to refrain from sex for the first three months because he wasn't too strong, but after that time, he could resume a normal sex life.

"Now everything is fine. I have more interest in sex now than before the transplant," he said.

Crosby is obviously thrilled with his restored health: "Look, there's nothing wrong with me now. I'm just like you. I have to take medication, but I'm as good as you. I hope a foundation can be started so other people can have transplants, too. It's very expensive after the transplant because of the medicine."

We had talked for more than an hour, and Crosby had to get to class.

"Good luck to you, Crosby," I said, as we shook hands and said goodbye. He disappeared out the door as quickly as he had come, with an air of purpose and enthusiasm.

I left the hospital shortly afterward, remembering Kelly's gentle honesty and Crosby's happy face.

Later that day, I called Mary Wilkerson, a recent transplant patient, and made an appointment for Saturday when we could meet and talk. I had learned that black people often waited longer for transplants than white people did, and I was interested in learning from Mary, who is black, if that had been her experience.

Mary, Ardelle, and I were to have dinner. A half-hour after the time of our appointment, Mary called. "Pat, this is Mary. I've had a car accident and I'm going to the hospital to be checked. I want to be sure nothing's happened to my heart."

I told her to call as soon as she could to let me know how she was. I waited two hours and, finally, the phone rang. "I'm okay," Mary announced. "Can I still come and see you?"

"Oh, yes!" I told her, my spirits soaring with relief.

It was 9:30 P.M. when she arrived, walking gingerly into the room.

I hugged her carefully. "It looks like you're in pain," I said.

"I am, but not from the accident," she said.

"What's the matter?" I pursued.

"Well, to be perfectly frank, I have a severe case of genital warts. It's from the cyclosporine. I can hardly walk or sit down." She sat down, grimacing.

"I just learned today about that side-effect," I told her, remembering my conversation with Kelly.

The hotel restaurant was just closing as we arrived, but the staff there agreed to serve us anyway. Mary hadn't brought her medicine, thinking she'd be home before she needed to take it, so she shared Ardelle's cyclosporine, mixed with orange juice. It was nice to have no other diners around so we could talk freely. I turned on the tape recorder and Mary began to tell us her story.

Mary's heart problem first surfaced as exhaustion: "I'd come home from work and go to bed early. Then I'd wake up feeling as if I'd never gotten any sleep. I thought there was something wrong because I'm usually a very energetic person. So I went to see a doctor. He said I had tonsillitis and gave me some pills, but they didn't work.

"I was still feeling tired, so I went to another doctor. I had had a cold for a long time and it wouldn't go away. The doctor took a chest x-ray and wanted to put me in the hospital immediately. I said, 'I can't do that! What's wrong with me anyway?' He told me I had an enlarged heart.

"I went into the hospital the next day and remained there for two weeks," said Mary. "I lost twelve pounds in one day when they removed the fluid that had built up. The doctor came in and asked me if I had a will and I said I didn't. 'Well, I think it's time for you to make one out,' he told me. That really scared me.

"After I was feeling better, he sent me home, but he told me not to go back to work and to just take it very easy. So I stayed at home for a couple weeks and I got sick again. Then I was back in the hospital. From then on, I was back and forth to the hospital every few weeks. This all started in February of 1989, so I had to wait a whole year for the transplant.

"I had HMO insurance, and they wouldn't pay for a transplant, so I had to go back to work even though I was very sick. By doing that, I was able to switch my insurance in October to a company that covered transplants. I tried to work for two weeks, but I couldn't make it. The ambulance had to come and get me at work and take me back to the hospital.

"The new insurance didn't go into effect until January first, so I had to wait some more. But at least I was on the list as of the first of the year.

"Shortly before my new heart arrived, I moved into another apartment so I could be closer to the hospital. My phone wasn't installed yet, but the transplant office had my friend, Mark St. John's number to call until my phone was in. Mark helped me move, and then we went out to eat, but I was really tired and I decided to go home and take a hot bath and relax.

"All of a sudden I heard someone knocking on the door. I looked out the bedroom window and there were Mark and Terry, another friend of mine. I yelled out the window, 'Just a minute.' I grabbed a bathrobe and let them in. 'I'm just taking a bath," I said. 'Make yourselves at home and I'll be done in a few minutes," and I headed back to the tub.

"But Mark couldn't wait to tell the news. 'Pat called,' he said. I said, 'What Pat?' 'Pat from the transplant office,' he answered. 'They have a heart for you.'

"I lost it right there. I had no control over my body and I started shaking. I knew the heart I had was no good, but you never know what you're going to get! I was a total basket case. We went to the gas station down the street and called the transplant office to let them know I'd take it anyway.

"Mark went home and called everybody I knew to tell them the good news. And he beat me to the hospital. That was the first time in his life he's ever been on time for anything!

"I was still scared to death, but I wasn't about to not get that heart, either. And by the time they did all the tests, and the surgery was done, it was my birthday. What a present!

"I stayed in the hospital two weeks. When I came home, I had no strength. I couldn't even pick up my purse. My hemoglobin was so low I needed a blood transfusion. I was really worried about that with the AIDS thing, but the doctors said they screen the blood very carefully.

"A few weeks after the transfusion, I started to reject. I had to go back in for three massive dosages of steroids to stop it. Since then, everything has been fine except for the side effects."

Mary's side effects haven't been easy to endure. She suffers from severe tremors and cramps. But for Mary, the genital warts have been the most painful and traumatic aspect of the aftermath. She had laser surgery for them and they came back, more severe than ever.

She has suffered from extreme depression, too, and said that's a sharp contrast from her usual bright outlook on life. But her changed physical appearance, including her puffy face, has no doubt contributed to her gloomy moods. She lost all her hair as a result of having a permanent wave after the transplant. But it's back now and looking beautiful. In contrast, she's had excessive hair growth all over the rest of her body.

"It's really bad, especially for a lady. We're not supposed to have mustaches and hairy arms," she laughed.

Mary doesn't plan to go back to her previous job because it was very stressful. But she's worried about getting another one. She sees some things in her favor, however.

"I'm a black female, and now I'm classified as disabled, too," she laughed. "I know I have to get a job with a big company so I have good insurance. I don't plan to offer the information that I've had a transplant, but I know I'll be asked if I take any drugs, so I'll have to list those, and that's quite a list!"

In response to my concerns about racial bias in receiving a transplant, she said: "I can't say that anyone discriminated against me or anyone else at the transplant office. I don't think black people know about transplants as they should. I saw on TV that the rate of black people who donate organs is very low for the simple reason that we don't know enough about transplants. And we don't know people who have had them. Some of my friends said that just to look at me now, they would be willing to donate their organs."

Mary's friends have been a vital link to her recovery, and she's gotten a lot of support from the transplant program, too. "They really care about me. Even the chief surgeon, Dr. Ring, remembers me and always stops to talk," she said.

But financial problems have hounded her. She received disability payments of $150 a week for 26 weeks from her employer. That paid the rent and some of the utilities.

"I went through some very, very hard times—the worst of my life—but I made it. I'm still going through some hard times. I get $760 a month from Social Security Disability, but when your rent is $400 and utilities are $313, you have nothing left. There's still car insurance and all the other things you need. If it hadn't been for my friends, I don't know how I would have made it," she recalled.

Despite the problems, Mary said, without hesitation, she would go through another transplant if something went wrong with this heart and another was offered. She isn't to the point yet, however, where she feels her life is back to normal.

"I have no control over my life yet. The transplant office and the medication control my life—and I resent that. I had always controlled my life before, but don't misunderstand me. I'm very grateful and very blessed to have had such a good medical team," she added.

She had some words of advice for potential transplant patients: "Be ready to go through all the changes your body will take you through, because there are many of them. You have to sacrifice. You're going to hear 'do this, do that, don't do this, don't do that.' But hang in there because things get better as time goes by."

Guidepost: Learning as We Go

Meeting with Kelly in Dallas proved to be a highlight of my research on transplants. Her candid discussion of both the positive and negative sides of the issue helped me understand the wide range of concerns recipients share. I had sometimes found a reluctance on the part of staff members to talk about the down side. Yet I knew it was there. Kelly seemed to understand that the more information a recipient has, the easier the adjustment to a new lifestyle.

I encourage prospective recipients and their families to ask every question that comes to mind. If the staff members don't know the answers, ask them to find out for you. You are in the process of making one of the most important decisions of your life, and you deserve to know every aspect of it.

11

Robert: Unexpected Roadblocks

Robert Dobberpuhl of Cedarburg, Wisconsin, is alive and full of energy at the age of 28. At 5-feet, 11-inches tall, and weighing 170 pounds, he has the body of a disciplined athlete. His stamina in running, playing tennis, basketball, and volleyball, along with biking and weight-lifting, makes him the envy of his friends. He's an inspiring role model for other kidney transplant recipients. But he's caught in a trap that has derailed a dream.

"I've recently experienced one of the most profound disappointments of my life," he said. "When I received my transplant, I was completing work for my master's degree in history, and it's been my greatest dream since that time to go back to school and get my Ph.D.

"Earlier this year, I was accepted by two major universities and offered substantial fellowship money by both schools to study for my degree. I scored in the top 6 percent nationally on my graduate record exams. But neither school's health insurance would cover the cost of my drugs. I spoke with individuals associated with every social help organization and government agency I could think of. I wrote to one of my senators, with whose help I pursued more organizations and ideas.

"But nothing worked. All of the programs were useless to me and my future. Since then I've been wondering why my hopes and dreams have been derailed," Robert said.

He believes a national program to assist inadequately insured transplant recipients in covering the cost of drugs would put his life on track again. Now he feels trapped in his job where his health insurance picks up much of the cost. "Before I can even think of changing jobs or trying to improve myself, I have to worry about how I'll pay for my drugs. Mine total about $700 a month, so without adequate health insurance, while my friends bought houses, I'd be buying the right to stay alive and off dialysis," he explained.

Recently Robert suffered another financial blow. His employer switched insurance companies, and Robert was told he would have to pay up-front for his drugs and then be reimbursed by the insurer, placing him in a position of buying his drugs or paying his rent. His pharmacist, aware of Robert's financial burdens, agreed to let him have a pharmacy charge card, and he will be able to pay after he's reimbursed. But the experience has angered Robert. It reminds him once again how very vulnerable he is.

"My big question now is whether I have much of a future to look forward to," he said. "With my company's change in insurance, I can look forward to some wonderful financial problems. But I have no choice. I've already resolved that I'll do whatever it takes to keep my kidney. If I have to break into pharmacies and simply take the medications I need, I'll do so without feeling any guilt. Maybe that's what it will take to have the lethargic people in this country wake up and understand what some of us have to go through. It's a matter of life and death for me, so society's rules just don't apply anymore. Perhaps my only choice is to leave this country and go to one that offers a national health program that will allow me to live my life as I wish.

"I don't think I've ever been so full of anger and frustration in my life. My transplant has been one long miserable experience. It has even influenced my relationship with a woman I love. She wonders how financially secure she can ever be with someone who has to take $700 worth of medication a month and can't get adequate insurance. So what, if anything, do I really have to look forward to?" he asked.

Robert lost his second kidney in 1987, at the age of 25. His first kidney had been removed in 1984 as one of the tragic effects of a genetic disorder, von Hippel-Lindau's syndrome. His father, his father's three brothers, and a cousin have died from the disease that causes tumors of the kidney, pancreas, cerebellum, retina, and spine. Robert has suffered from tumors in most of those areas except the spine.

Two of his four sisters also have von Hippel-Lindau's syndrome. One has undergone numerous retinal surgeries and two brain surgeries and has lost one of her kidneys. There are cysts on the remaining kidney, and she may face a transplant in the future. Another sister has had surgery for a spinal tumor, which has recently recurred.

The effects of Robert's disease surfaced when he was 14. He suffered headaches, nausea, and dizziness, and doctors diagnosed his first brain tumor. At 16, he had laser surgery on his left eye after a retinal angioma was found. Two years later, cysts were found in both kidneys. At 21, when the first nephrectomy was done, doctors found 19 tumors in the kidney.

Then, when his second kidney was removed, three years later, he was placed on dialysis. "I knew I wanted a transplant as soon as I had gone through my first day without any kidneys," he said. "I was frequently sick and had only enough energy to make it through half a day before I had to take a nap. I didn't like the idea of being dependent on medications for the rest of my life, but it seemed a small price to pay compared with being hooked up to a dialysis machine three days a week.

"Several friends offered their kidneys, but their blood types didn't match. My wife, at the time, offered to donate because her blood type did match, and she began the tests necessary to determine if other factors were compatible. They were, and we went ahead with the transplant in February 1988, even though I felt very guilty about her decision. I knew it wouldn't be easy, and I had tried on several occasions to talk her out of it.

"After the surgery, we were placed on opposite ends of the hospital wing, and we'd have to walk to see each other. I felt very sorry for her because she didn't recover very quickly. She was in a lot of pain, and it hurt me to know that she had done what she had for my sake. Our marriage had not been a happy one, and we had considered divorce after my second nephrectomy.

"Our marriage improved for a while after the transplant, but it didn't last. I think my new chance to live made me realize I had been wasting my life."

That emotional stress is only one side effect of the transplant. Robert has also suffered others, such as acne on his back, shoulders, upper arms, and chest, especially in the summer when he's active outdoors. His face is a little fatter, he says, but he's happy he can finally grow a full beard and even a few chest hairs!

In the first month after transplantation, he gained 20 pounds because he could eat all the foods denied him while on dialysis. But after he resumed his exercise schedule, he lost the weight over a period of three and a half years.

His diet, he knows, is one that most transplant doctors would not condone. "I live on sugar—doughnuts, cookies, soda, and candy bars. But I also sneak in a few steaks, some fish, some fruit, a glass of wine now and then, and an occasional potato. Vegetables in general are lacking from my diet because, well, I just don't like them and never did!" he explained.

He says his mood swings are more dramatic than before, but he admits to always having been a little "high strung." In fact, a girl friend characterized him as a "coiled spring," and he thinks that fits.

His sex life hasn't been impaired. The sexual relationship between him and his wife improved for a few months after the transplant, and since his divorce, he's had other intimate relationships that have been intense.

"When I was 18, I thought the best thing that could happen to me would be to meet a nymphomaniac; now that I'm 28, I still feel the same way," he laughed, his bright blue eyes twinkling.

But behind the sparkle, there is still the frustration of a young man with unfulfilled dreams that seem to drift further and further away. And he asks some questions he would like answered. "Does it make any sense that doctors can offer us the chance at a renewed life via a transplant, only to have society close off jobs and opportunities to us? What about those who can't find affordable insurance and simply cease taking their medications when Medicare coverage expires?

Must we spend the rest of our lives paying for the right to be alive?

"It's time we begin to raise our voices on this issue. We need to write to our representatives in Washington and to the President himself, demanding a national program be initiated to assist transplantees with the cost of their drugs.

"I'd hoping to circulate petitions to this effect among transplant facilities nationwide. I think we need to push this issue because if we don't, no one else will," he said.

Guidepost: Finding the Money

Money is always a concern for the transplant patient. Even the most generous insurance plans often impose lifetime caps—and these are well within the reach of many transplantees. As Robert explains, some of the laws governing who and what is paid for are not based on the most logical decision making.

Each of us needs to be aware of exactly what kind of insurance we have and what is covered and what isn't. And we need to use our insurance benefits as wisely as possible.

Most transplant centers have social workers to help work through financial problems. Soon many will also have financial advisers to assist with insurance and other financial concerns. Being aware of the help and options available to you is an important part of handling the stress that money problems trigger.

Find a support group and get involved in it. They are invariably a rich source of information on all aspects of transplant life.

12

Rick: A Donor Family's Tragedy

Author's Note: *The following three chapters deal with the subject of organ donation. The names of the hospitals where the donations were made are not included because it is not my goal to place blame on or to praise any institution. Rather it is to provide insight and information with the hope that sensitivity to donor needs will be improved.*

When 16-year-old Rick Kangas took a class on death and dying, he laid the foundation for life, built upon his tragic accidental death less than a year later.

That class was held in the fall of 1977. Teacher and students visited local cemeteries and talked about donating organs, something that was new and controversial. In 1976, a family friend who died of cancer had donated her body to the University of Minnesota for study. Those two events had made an indelible impression on Rick.

At a Thanksgiving gathering in 1977, he told his family that if he should die, he wanted his organs donated so others could live. But who could even imagine this young, bright-eyed kid with the effervescent smile being anything but alive and happy and going places.

Certainly not his mother, Phyllis Lamkin of Burnsville, Minnesota, who had bought him a motorcycle to fulfill one of his boyhood dreams. He had met and spent time with Evel Knevel, a daredevil motorcyclist who had warned Rick to never try any stunts and to always wear a helmet when he rode his bike.

Rick usually lived by that advice. But one July evening in 1976 he was just going to the schoolyard down the block to play basketball with his friends. One of his buddies was there with his cycle, too, and Rick didn't put his helmet on when the two began an impromptu Evel Knevel trick.

They started down a driveway, then stood up on the seat of their motorcycles, arms outstretched, with a group of friends watching. Just as Rick was about to sit down, the front wheel of his bike hit a stone and flipped Rick backwards. He hit the base of his head, staggered to his feet and collapsed. "Get my Mom," he said.

Rick suffered a severe brain stem injury, and doctors at a local hospital saw no indication of life from the EEG they administered. His family waited, in shock. There was no bruise, no bleeding. It looked to his 11-year-old brother as though Rick was just asleep.

Both his mom, Phyllis, and his sister, Debbie, recall that no doctor ever took the time to talk to the family. All the information they received came through a nurse. And when the final EEG was given to Rick, 14 hours after the accident, Phyllis stood outside the hospital curtain waiting for the results. As the doctor swished the curtain aside and came out laughing and talking to another doctor, she was convinced that miraculously, Rick must have recovered. The doctor brushed past her without a word and she rushed toward her son's bed. Then she saw the nurse standing beside him, sobbing.

"Why are you crying? He's all right, isn't he?" Phyllis asked.

The nurse shook her head. "No," she said through her tears. "I'm sorry. He's brain dead."

"The nurses did their best to comfort us," Phyllis said. "They explained how the brain wave tests were done and that after three flat tests, a person is declared legally dead. I wish a doctor had explained to us more thoroughly how they came to that conclusion. There were no outward signs of injury, and it was almost impossible for us to accept it."

During that long night of waiting, Phyllis and her five remaining children remembered Rick's request to donate his organs. They made the decision to honor his wish, which had seemed so remote that Thanksgiving afternoon.

"At that time the hospital didn't have any donor forms so, after the final EEG, the nurse called the University of Minnesota Hospital and they dictated the forms over the phone. We donated his heart, his pancreas, liver, kidneys, and corneas. We didn't know it at the time, but Sue Huff of Baxter, Minnesota, was near death from a heart disease. She was waiting for a transplant and Rick's heart was a perfect match. By coincidence, my father had known Sue's husband, Bob, for many years," Phyllis said.

His other organs were transplanted, too. Phyllis recalls that his pancreas was the first one ever transplanted, and the recipient's life was turned around, making an amazing recovery from her diabetes.

Phyllis said that everyone was okay with the donation except Rick's dad, from whom she is divorced.

"He didn't know Rick's wishes because he wasn't living with the family then," Phyllis said. "And he's still not convinced that Rick was dead when his organs were removed. Again, if the doctor had taken the time to help him understand the process, it could have been easier on him."

Debbie, Rick's sister, agreed with donating Rick's organs but isn't comfortable with the fact that her mother became friends with Sue Huff, the woman who received Rick's heart. Phyllis and Sue have appeared on TV programs and radio talk shows to promote donor awareness and have gone to Disney World together to celebrate life.

"I don't want to know Sue," Debbie said. "I'm glad she's doing fine, but I would never have known her if Rick hadn't died, so I don't want to know her. It bothers me when my mom spends time with her, but I know it helps my mom."

But in her own way, Debbie promotes donor awareness too. She was interviewed by a local newspaper, and she's given speeches and written papers about the experience. But there often seems to be a negative.

"After an article appeared in the newspaper, someone said to me, 'Gee, some people will do anything to get in the paper,'" Debbie said.

Phyllis and Debbie believe that writing and speaking about the experience is a way to process the grief. Debbie admits she held her feelings in for years: "I didn't cry at the funeral or afterwards. Then one day two years later, I was coming home from work, and I started to cry. All of a sudden, it just came out."

Phyllis finds that being part of Sue's life gives her some peace after a long, terrible struggle with guilt and debilitating grief. Part of the guilt centered on her having bought the motorcycle for Rick just ten days before the accident.

"There were days that I didn't think I could get through. I wanted to kill myself," Phyllis said.

"We received hate mail and phone calls after news got out that we had donated Rick's organs. That was really hard on the family. We thought we had done a good thing, and these anonymous letters told us that unless he was saved by Jesus, he'd go to Hell no matter what good things he'd done. Then a relative told us that if Rick hadn't been a Catholic, he wouldn't have died. I felt like I was going crazy. All these terrible things were happening.

"I went to a grief counselor someone recommended, and she really saved my life. There weren't any donor family support groups, so I was on my own. Sometimes I could just barely drag myself out my door to go see her, and when I'd get there, I'd say, 'Today I could have run into a bridge abutment or into another car, but I didn't.' She understood exactly what I was telling her. She turned things around and helped me realize how lucky we were to have had Rick for 16 wonderful years. 'You could have gone through your life without ever knowing him,' she told me."

Inadvertently Rick also left his mother some consolation. Phyllis described it this way: "After he died, I didn't touch anything of his for over a year. Before the accident, he was supposed to go in for surgery on his back. He had a slight curvature of the spine and that would mean being in a body cast for a year. So he had decided to go through all his papers and get rid of lots of stuff because he would have to live in that room for a year. I remember him carrying boxes of paper out to the trash. After he died, there wasn't much left.

"But I found one piece of paper with an American Indian poem he had copied. It was so beautiful. It goes like this:

> *Although I die, I shall continue*
> *to live in everything that is.*
> *The buffalo eats the grass.*
> *And I eat him; and when I die,*
> *the earth eats me and sprouts more grass.*
> *Therefore, nothing is ever lost*
> *and each thing is everything forever."*

Phyllis believes organized support for donor families is missing from many transplant situations. And Debbie believes doctors should be required to take sensitivity classes to help them better understand the emotions surrounding sudden death, donation, and transplantation.

"They need to understand that's part of their job. Nurses shouldn't be the only caregivers. The doctor should sit and talk and give the facts and then help the family process through the immediate crisis. In our situation, the doctor was so insensitive it was hard to believe he was even on the case," she said.

Phyllis and Debbie are convinced that donor family needs aren't addressed because hospital staffs think of the donor's death as a stepping stone to the transplant procedure and not an end in itself. While Phyllis and Debbie understand the importance of the transplant, they also understand when they hear donor families say they felt "in the way."

"I believe one specific person should be assigned to a donor family and should stay with them throughout the process. That issue just has to be addressed," Debbie said.

"There's also the issue of brain death and how it's determined. I've had many people ask me, 'Was your brother really dead?' And after a while, you begin to wonder about it yourself. Especially when you hear of people who've been in a coma for years and suddenly wake up," Debbie said.

Phyllis recalled that when Rick died, brain death was still a very controversial issue. And she remembers that Rick's temperature was high and his pulse erratic. Otherwise, he looked fine.

"My son, 11-year-old Jamie, said, 'Why are they going to kill him? He just has to wake up.' If the doctor had come in and explained things to us, we probably would have dealt with it better as a family. Most people accept the doctor as the final authority, and that was the missing link for us," Phyllis said.

"No one explained how the organs were taken or if there was any anesthesia used or if he could have felt anything. I've asked myself these questions through the years, and so has my dad," Debbie said.

"Another thing they failed to tell us about, which was a real shock," Debbie said, "was what kind of condition Rick would be in afterwards. When we saw him again at the church we didn't recognize him.

"He was twice his normal size because of the drugs and the process used to keep his organs functioning. He had been a slim, trim young man who was very conscious of his appearance. Between the mortician fixing his hair wrong and then seeing him so bloated, we were horrified. Had we known how he would look, we would have had a closed casket."

"The minute I saw him," Phyllis said, "I just shut myself off. I couldn't believe it was him. I thought, 'Why are we all here? That isn't Rick.' I just wanted to get out of there."

Since the nightmare of her son's death, Phyllis finds it healing to concentrate as much as possible on the miracle of life the donation offered. It gives her joy to know Sue, who is the longest living transplant patient in Minnesota, and to know that the other recipients of Rick's organs are doing well, too.

"Many miracles came from his donation. I'm proud of my son who was such a thoughtful, generous young man in life as well as in death," Phyllis said.

Debbie finds comfort in that, too, but from a distance. She's listed as a donor even though her husband and children don't like the idea very much. In that regard, she's very like her mother who says, "If you have something that someone can use, you shouldn't throw it away."

Rick believed that, too.

13

Bob: Unacknowledged Grief

Jan and Bob Dale of Kensington, Minnesota, had planned to go to Minneapolis for the weekend to attend the races at the local track. Instead, Jan and her three grown children faced Bob's sudden death and the decision to donate his organs at a Twin Cities hospital. His death was traumatic and shocking. The donation of his organs was so painful for the family that three years later, they still find no consolation in it.

The Dales believe from the moment they signed the donation papers, their feelings became irrelevant. They believe they were shoved aside, ignored, and in the way. They believe the medical system, with its state-of-the-art technology, failed them as grieving, stunned human beings who had lost a family member.

Jan tells their story, not to discourage other families from participating in the organ donor program, but to encourage medical facilities to look at how they can best meet the needs of people who wish, in their own devastating loss, to give the gift of life.

"It's in the hospitals' best interest. The hospitals need the donor organs. I know my family's experience has turned off some people who had considered being donors. That could mean that people on the waiting list will die for lack of those organs," Jan said.

The Dale family's ordeal began as an ordinary day on July 1, 1988. Jan and Bob awoke at 5:30 A.M., and Jan went to the kitchen to make coffee. She was on summer vacation from her teaching job but Bob needed to be at work at the print shop by 6:30. After work the two of them planned to leave for the Twin Cities for a weekend of fun. They were a close-knit family with a love for hunting together in the woodlands of central Minnesota. Now that the children were grown and gone from home, Jan and Bob were enjoying a new freedom.

The first rays of morning sun touched the window as Jan measured the coffee and began the morning breakfast ritual. Then she heard Bob call her name and the normality of the day came to an unexpected end.

"I went in to see what he wanted," Jan said. "He was vomiting and he said, 'Something's happened. I can't feel my legs.'

"I called First Responders and then helped Bob get dressed. He was still nauseated and had a terrible headache. I thought maybe he'd had a seizure or a stroke. I sat by the bed and talked to him while we waited for the ambulance. He looked up at me and said, 'Jan, I love you but I'm dying.'

"Of course, I didn't believe that. He was kind of a wimp when it came to medical things. He hated doctors and hospitals and over-reacted to a headcold," Jan said. Still she remembers thinking, as she followed the ambulance to the hospital, "I'm too young for this." Bob was just 47 and she was 46.

"There was no doctor on duty when we got there," Jan said, "and Bob lay in the emergency room for 40 minutes without treatment. But he was lucid and talked to us and I thought everything would be all right. My older son John was with me and that helped tremendously. We called the other kids. Debbie was in Minneapolis and Danny was attending college.

"Bob kept complaining about his awful headache. When the doctor finally arrived and examined Bob, he told me, 'Jan, Bob has either an aneurysm or an embolism and we won't know which unless we do a spinal tap.'

"At that point, if they had asked me to cut off my legs I would have done it. I signed the paper to have it done," Jan said.

"Our family doctor, who was leaving on vacation, stopped in to see his patients before leaving town, and he saw Bob, too. He told me Bob was critical. I knew that was bad but I didn't know critical meant you could die," she said. "But while we were talking I heard the code and I knew what it was. Bob had arrested during the spinal tap."

Suddenly a flurry of people rushed into Bob's room. They were able to resuscitate him and get him on a respirator while Jan and John, in shocked disbelief, stood trembling in the hall.

"The doctor told us Bob needed to be transported to another hospital, and we chose one in Minneapolis. I called Bob's parents and other family members while we waited for the helicopter. I couldn't fly with him, so John and I headed for Minneapolis in Danny's old beater car that Bob had been working on.

"We didn't say much on the way down. We didn't talk about what we'd do if he died or anything like that. We just talked about whom we had contacted and whom we needed to contact," Jan recalled.

Debbie and her husband met the helicopter when it arrived at the hospital and were the first family members to be told the tragic news that nothing could be done to save Bob's life.

Grief-stricken, they met Jan and John at the hospital after their long and nerve-wracking drive from Kensington. Jan folded Debbie into her arms as Debbie sobbed out the awful news. It was as if the world had stopped on that July morning and it would never again go on as it had.

Jan remembers that people came from all over—Danny, brothers and sisters, cousins, parents, friends. An intern pastor at the hospital was with them, getting coffee and making phone calls. Family members took turns going into Bob's room to watch for some small sign of hope, but there was none.

One of the nurses had told Debbie to keep talking to him because, she said, hearing is the last sense to go. So Debbie talked and talked, telling her father over and over again that she loved him; stroking his face and his silver-blond hair. No one told her to stop, and she kept on.

Sometime in that unbelievable afternoon a doctor told them Bob was brain dead. He had suffered an intracranial hemorrhage.

"He told us he had no response to pain tests and my imagination went wild," Jan said. "I saw eight-foot-long needles in his brain. But I didn't ask what they had done and no one told me. Later I learned the test is very simple—merely pressing beneath the breastbone. I wish they had explained that to me and not let me imagine those horrible things. I wish they had at least asked me if I wanted to know how the testing was done.

"I asked how long Bob could live on a respirator and the doctor said, 'He has a strong heart. He could live for days, months, years.' I knew Bob wouldn't want to be kept alive if things couldn't be reversed. I knew how he hated hospitals."

As Jan recalls, it was Bob's mother who brought up the subject of donating his organs. It was something Bob had never expressed his wishes about, although he knew Jan was listed as a donor.

"The doctor said he'd send someone to talk to us about it," Jan said. "But first the children and I wanted to discuss it privately, so we went off by ourselves to another room. While we were there, Bob's nurses came in. One of the children asked her if we could be with Bob when he died. She said that, yes, we could be with him when they took him off the respirator so that he could die with us around him, and then they would harvest the organs. My sister and I knew that wasn't correct.

"Up to that point, the children were 100 percent for the donation as long as we could be with him when they took him off the respirator. After the nurse left, my sister looked at me and said, 'I know that's not right. Let me get the head nurse so that we can be clear about this.'

"The head nurse explained that Bob would have to be on the respirator when the organs were removed in order to keep the organs functioning.

"That's when the trouble started.

"Debbie said, 'If Dad's got to die, I want to be with him.' John was still in favor of the donation, and Danny wasn't saying. It got real bad between the children, so we decided to talk to the rest of the family. Bob's dad was against it, too, if he had to be kept on the respirator.

"About that time, Bob's brother arrived. Everybody expressed opinions, and I tried to consider all of them. I wanted to work something out so everyone would accept it. The kids started yelling and screaming and swearing at each other. It was just the most awful thing. Of all the things that happened that day, that was the second worst.

"Because Bob had never expressed any wishes about being a donor, we talked about the kind of person he was. He was helping people all the time, and I'd get angry about it. I'd say, 'Why don't you stay home and put on your own storm windows instead of going over and shingling the neighbor's roof?' 'But helping people makes me feel good,' he'd say.

"But even after remembering those things, it was obvious I'd never get a consensus. I went off with the transplant coordinator and the intern pastor to make a decision on my own. I had a lot of questions. And I needed to know what would happen and the timelines around which I'd have to make decisions about the funeral. They were both supportive and helpful, and I decided I'd go ahead. I told them, 'I know the children are angry, but they love me and will accept my decision.'

"I checked the organs he'd donate and signed the donor paper. I also signed a paper stipulating that Bob's body would be taken to the mortuary in Morris, Minnesota. Then I made the children sign the donation paper, too. 'This is what we're going to do, and we're going to do it as a family,' I told them.

"Up to that point, I felt everyone had been wonderful—except for the nurse who gave us the wrong information. But then the procedure started to fall apart. From the moment we signed the paper, we felt everything changed. It was as if they'd gotten what they wanted and we were merely in the way.

"They said they'd need to run some tests that would take only a little while, and then we could spend all the time we wanted with him.

"That short period of time stretched into hours. People were coming and going into his room hauling equipment in and out. When we asked how much longer we'd have to wait, it was always 'just a little longer,'" Jan recalled.

Four hours passed. No one from the medical staff came to talk to the family and they believed they were given only evasive answers to questions. Somewhere in there, Jan recalls, a doctor came out and asked her if Bob smoked. She assumed they were thinking of a heart-lung transplant. But there were no words of consolation, no acknowledgment of the horrible thing they were going through, and no words of thanks for the gracious gift. There was no offer of a bowl of soup or cup of coffee. They were irrelevant, Jan felt.

"Finally the coordinator came to us and told us testing was done and we could go back in. He said that when we were finished, they'd take Bob into surgery and harvest the organs and should be done by 3:00 A.M. We went back in and said our last good-byes, and sometime after midnight we left," Jan said.

At noon the next day, Jan returned home to a jangling phone. It was the mortician from Morris, a friend of the family's.

"What happened to Bob?" he asked.

"He died," Jan told him.

"People have been calling here asking when the funeral will be and I haven't heard from the hospital," he said.

"I signed the paper at the hospital telling them which mortuary they should take him to. I assumed they would call and make arrangements, but obviously they haven't done that. I'll call the hospital to see what happened," she told the mortician.

"My hands were shaking as I dialed the phone. I was so angry. When I got hold of the right person at the hospital, I was told that things were taking longer than they thought and the body might be ready to be released by three o'clock that afternoon. They said they'd notify the mortuary then. I was just furious. Just furious.

"I found out later that my daughter-in-law had called the hospital at six that morning, and they were just taking Bob into the operating room then. He'd been on the respirator all night and we thought it was over. I resent that. I think they should have been in touch with me to say, 'Things are taking longer than we thought. If you want to come back and spend more time with him, you're free to do that.'

"As it was, we had felt pressure to be done and to leave when they said the surgery would be completed by three in the morning. They shouldn't have let us think that it was over and he was at peace when they hadn't even taken him into the damned operating room. I've never gotten an explanation that satisfies me.

"It was a holiday weekend, they said, and they were short-staffed. But I said, 'Hey, holiday weekends are great opportunities. Lots of people die in accidents.'

"They said the cross-matching took longer than expected. The woman who got Bob's heart had antigens that were difficult to match. The liver transplant team from Chicago was late in arriving, they told me.

"Maybe I could have accepted those explanations if they had communicated with me. If they had given me some input into the process, I might feel differently. But I felt, and the kids felt too, that the moment we signed that paper he was theirs. Whatever we were feeling or whatever part we played in his life or in his dying wasn't important anymore.

"As it was, his body didn't arrive at the mortuary until Saturday, 20 hours after his death, and the funeral was on Tuesday.

"Within the week I started getting the bills. I had been told that once the paper was signed, all expenses of harvesting the organs became the recipient's. But the Notice of Resolution of $13,782 from the insurance company still left a balance of $4,259. That seemed very high for seven hours of hospitalization.

"I called the hospital and asked for an itemized bill. It didn't arrive until weeks later and it had some strange and unusual dates on it. Bob died on the first of July and some dates were for the sixth. One was for an anesthesiologist and I couldn't understand why they needed that for a dead man. I eventually discovered that I'd been billed for about $10,000 of recipient charges.

"I had also spent hundreds of dollars for phone calls and written volumes of letters trying to resolve these misunderstandings. Once when I called the hospital about the bill, I was asked, 'Why should this be a concern to you? The insurance company is paying for it.' I said, 'We all pay for it through increased premiums.'

"The aftermath was almost worse than his dying. The hospital did apologize for the problems we had, and they settled for the insurance company's check as payment in full. But it took months to get it all straightened out. Bob died in July, and by Christmas I was having such a stressful time that my doctor wanted to hospitalize me, but I said no. He convinced me then to take time from my job to get everything resolved, which I did. By having good intentions we caused ourselves a tremendous amount of pain. And it still goes on.

I think to myself, 'I should be happy that we helped others to live' but I'm not. We received a letter from the heart recipient, and my daughter won't even look at it. One night when her husband was on a hunting trip, she came to see me and we talked most of the night. She was still deeply troubled by what happened. But she's come to the point where she can say, 'Mom, you've made a lot of other decisions for me, and they were right. I have to believe that this was right, too.'"

Jan's rage is over, but her anger and resentment still smoulder. From a distance of time, she can analyze what went wrong. And she hopes that, through her story, hospitals will make some changes in their approach to donor families.

"If a hospital is going to have a donor program, they need a donor family support group. It would have been so helpful for us if someone from a donor family could have been with us through this terrible ordeal. And afterwards we could go to them and ask for help with things such as the billing. I've never met another donor family, and I feel very isolated. I went in search of a grief support group and have tried to help myself as much as I can, but I was offered nothing at the time of Bob's death.

"Hospital staff need to be aware that this is a family that has just lost a loved one through a traumatic and sudden illness or accident. They're dealing with someone who has had no expectation or thoughts about being faced with this dilemma. They need to be there to walk us through it—because we've not walked there before and they have. They should make it their business to know what we need at that time because we don't know. They need to acknowledge that the family is going through a terrible, terrible experience.

"Perhaps acknowledgment is the biggest thing. The only person who ever said, 'This is horrible' was a counselor I went to. Up to that time, I had only heard that this was God's will, and to think of the good I did by donating his organs. No one said, 'This is just dreadful.' I remember feeling such relief when the counselor said that to me.

"And they need to use terminology that is understandable. They need to explain what 'critical' means. They need to at least ask a family how many details they want to know about determining brain death and how the organ harvesting is done.

"I also encourage people to talk about being a donor so that family members know their wishes. If the children and I had known Bob's wishes, it would have been so much easier.

"My daughter was listed as a donor before Bob's death, but she isn't now. My older son still is, but my younger son is not," she said.

Despite the aftermath, Jan is still registered as a donor. Before she went to London in 1990 on a grant for the National Foundation for the Humanities, she wrote a living will and put her affairs in order. "I didn't want my kids to have to go through this again," she said.

14

Mary and Tom:
Keepers of the Bridge

After talking with Jan Dale, I called the transplant program director at the hospital where the donation had been made and asked if I could talk to her about the Dale family experience. *Mary* (not her real name) offered to contact the transplant donor coordinator who had been involved so he could share his view of that event. I'll call him *Tom*.

The three of us met in a small office at the hospital. Both of them remembered well the tragic and traumatic experience the Dale family had gone through. And they were aware the family felt anger toward the hospital, believing the staff had been insensitive toward them.

While both maintain the procedure they followed during that family tragedy was the same one they used with other donor families, they are acutely aware that the experience for each family is horrendous.

"I think you can imagine. In their case, the Dales had planned to be off for the weekend. Within a matter of 48 hours, all your dreams are just shattered. All the plans for the next day and the rest of your life are gone. Jan had some tough decisions to make," Mary said.

"Jan was pretty strong about wanting to donate Bob's organs and she felt the children, even though they were angry, would get over it because they loved her and this was the right decision," she remembered.

"Their situation highlights the fact that none of us knows whether we'll be here tomorrow. But if you have the opportunity to decide what will happen to your organs, let your family know. That makes the decision a lot easier."

Tom added that *he* strives for unanimity among family members about whether or not a donation should be made. "But sometimes you're caught between a rock and a hard place when there's disagreement," he said. "The spouse, in this case, had the ultimate authority to make the decision, even though some of the children had reservations about it. But what you end up with are negative feelings that lie on the surface for a long time.

"Families in discord about the donation probably require a different approach than may have been made with the Dale family. Perhaps the better decision would have been to not donate at all. The pain of deciding may have caused more family strife than had they not donated. And perhaps that should have been the recommendation to them.

"We learned a lot from that experience. Now we want to make sure we clarify where the family is at. Do they understand that the patient has died? What had the doctor told them? What have other people told them about the process? There needs to be a careful exploration of the emotional issues around donation. The subject should be brought up only after the physician has come in and said the patient has died," he said.

"In this case," Tom recalled, "family members were arriving at different points, with different expectations. Some were dealing with a death and others were still dealing with the shock of an illness. And here's an organ coordinator talking about donation. Some family members may always wonder if donation was the right decision."

"Sudden death is traumatic enough, but then in the donor program, you're asked to stop in the midst of your own pain and think about someone else whom you can help to live. It's not an easy decision to make," Tom said.

I explained that the decision itself was only part of the unhappiness the family felt. Jan had said that once the donor organ paper was signed, the family believed they were pretty much ignored by the staff.

Tom explained the process he routinely followed at the hospital. "After the family has made their decision to donate, we offer the option to the family to stay, if they choose. But we usually encourage the family to go. Of course, we provide for them to spend time with their loved one to say good-bye. But things tend to get very busy once the donor papers are signed. Preparing for a donation is incredibly intensive and very, very time consuming. These patients have died. The bodily functions we take for granted are no longer working, and the caregivers are the brain for that person. We need to do a lot of things just to keep the organs functioning.

"Knowing all of this, I can understand where the family might feel neglected. It's probably accurate that we didn't spend much time with them. We were managing the decision-making process. The physicians come in and listen to the heart and make sure the kidneys and liver are functioning. We're scheduling surgery and trying to find recipients for those organs. All the organs have to have recipients lined up and the donor teams have to fly in all at the same time," Tom added.

Mary reminded me that a chaplain was with the Dales for much of the time, and she stressed that the staff tries to be sensitive to the family, allowing them to be together without a lot of interference. They had felt quite comfortable that at least one member of the staff was with the family, she said.

I told them Jan had, in retrospect, wished another donor family could have been with them for support. "Is that anything you'd consider as part of your program?" I asked.

Mary thought that might have helped the Dale family but others would resent strangers coming into such a personal tragedy. Even if a donor family had volunteered to do this, it would be difficult for them to go through that trauma again. "They would really have to be prepared to go back into that setting," she said.

Tom, too, had deep reservations about it: "I don't think, in my practice, that I'd do that. Both of those families would be at completely different emotional levels. I'm not sure we'd be prepared for the dynamics that might unfold. The whole donor issue is one that we really struggle with. We struggle between keeping them connected and letting them go to begin healing. It's a tough balancing act. How much time and attention do we provide these families? It's something we're all learning about, and it's an area that has gained a lot of organized thinking about what we should do.

"In my opinion, after working in this area now for six years, we should not be involved with them in any support or educational roles until they're out of their tragedy for at least two years. There's an awful lot of pain that goes on with the first birthday, the first holiday. But I do think there's value in making occasional phone calls to let them know we haven't forgotten them. I think there's a sense among donor families that they're sort of lost and forgotten. Everyone deals with their pain so individually that it's really difficult to fashion a bereavement support service."

"Some donor families write or call or say, 'It would really help me to know how the recipients are doing,'" Mary added. "But some of them have no desire to know anything about the recipient. They want to cut the strings and not be reminded of their tragedy."

Tom, now at a different facility, works with many families of children who have died. From that experience, he's rethinking the whole issue of whether a family should be encouraged to wait until the donation is complete and then see their family member again.

"Many families of children do that," he said, "and it may help them come to some closure. With adults, that often doesn't happen, and it's something we should be more sensitive to.

"If you think about it, the issues surrounding death in these patients has a visual conflict. When a person dies, there is no pulse, the chest is still, the flesh is cold, and there is a stillness about the patient. Intellectually and visually there's a connection. When patients die from an aneurysm and are on a ventilator, they die a neurological death and their bodily functions continue.

"We can tell the family the patient has died and intellectually the family believes us. But emotionally the family has not picked up the rest of it: the pulse that's still, the chest that is no longer rising and falling, the cold skin, the motionless heart monitor.

"The next time the family usually sees that patient is after the mortician has prepared the body for reviewal. They left the hospital with the intellectual knowledge but not the emotional connection. These are some of the things that we're learning in this very new field," Tom said.

I reminded them that in the Dale case, the family had been told they could be with Bob after he was taken off the respirator and before the organs were removed. That information was wrong, but it had helped the children accept the idea of donation, believing they could be with their dad free of all the machines and equipment. But when they learned that wasn't true, they reversed their decision. It seemed to me, that in their shock and grief, they were nonetheless aware of the need for closure that the coordinator talked about.

"I think we need to make the offer very clear to a family that they can stay and be with the patient after the surgery," Tom said. "We could find a quiet place where they can spend time with a husband or wife or child, and that may help. If my wife died, I think I would want to hold her even if there is no response. There's something about that final letting go that some donor families don't get."

I asked them about Jan's concern that the donation had taken place several hours later than the family had been told it would. And had they known that, they might have chosen to spend more time with Bob.

"Some of the problems were a result of misperceptions," Mary recalled. "Sometimes it's very hard for people to hear what they're being told during that moment of tremendous grief. And it's understandable that you're not going to listen to all the details.

"There were a few delays, and you can expect that to happen between midnight and six in the morning. Sometimes things just don't move as quickly then. Staffing was light in the lab, and the donor team couldn't get out of Chicago. We couldn't anticipate that," she said. "But we try to do the very best we can for the families."

Tom remembered that the surgery time change hadn't caused a funeral delay. If it had, he said he would have called the family right away to let them know. "Perhaps I should have called anyway, but I didn't," he said.

After we ended our conversation and said good-bye that afternoon, I walked back to my car, trying to sort everything out. I had been deeply touched by Jan Dale's painful story. Yet I had also felt pain in that small hospital conference room. It isn't an easy task to stand as the bridge between life and death, in an emotionally charged atmosphere where every action matters immensely.

This may be the most thankless part of the entire transplant procedure. Yet it's the vital link between the tragedy of sudden death and the wonder of renewed life. And it's a link that takes its own toll on those who must ask for the precious gift of donor organs while a family is facing its devastating loss.

In the process, the donor family needs on-going support, acknowledgment of their loss, and gratitude for their gift. In the activity that follows a donation, it's easy to see how the family might be neglected. Ensuring that doesn't happen should be as much a part of the procedure as all the other steps.

15

Juliette: Making Every Journey Count

Author's note: After reading the following letter from Juliette Exupery to Dr. David Lorber, I realized that it contained the bittersweet secret that makes organ donation a positive choice. That secret consists of a medical professional who deeply cares; one who is willing to educate a grief-stricken family about the procedure; and one who is able to help the family make a decision that will not only bring life to others, but that will bring a portion of consolation and peace to them.

My thanks to Juliette for allowing me to share her tribute with my readers.

Dear Dr. Lorber,

Some of us choose professions that do great service to mankind but, for the most part, are pretty thankless. I know: I've been a foster mother to 42 abused or abandoned children over the past eight years, and once in a while I long for just a little appreciation. It seldom comes. Your profession in service to others is similar. That's why I'm writing. Over the past 15 months I've had several opportunities to tell many people of the positive way in which you have influenced my life. I thought it was time I told you.

On November 6, 1988, you were given the grim task of examining, testing, and finally, pronouncing my daughter, Jamie, dead of carbon monoxide poisoning. She took her own life. Only God and Jamie know why. She was my only natural daughter and my best friend. She was 22 years old.

When you presented the opportunity for organ donation to our family, my initial response was swift and definite. I said, "I don't want my daughter chopped up." That could easily have been the end of the discussion. I have thanked you silently, and in public, many times since then for taking the issue one step further by saying, "Perhaps I could explain the surgical procedure to you." It was the word "surgical" that got my attention. I was picturing a "Jekyll and Hyde" laboratory with body parts in buckets. How easy it is for the imagination of the uneducated to erroneously influence major decisions.

During the brief explanation, you used words like reverence, dignity, and prosthetic replacement to restore the body for a normal burial. Most of all, you kept saying "Jamie." You didn't say "her" or "the patient" or "your loved one." I will never forget the sensitivity with which you explained the procurement procedures to us and answered our every question. In the end I voted with Jamie's three brothers that there was no reason not to donate. In our darkest hour you chose not to be intimidated by my initial response, nor did you retreat, as a physician with less courage might have. The result was that our family elected to make Jamie a full organ donor and that simple act changed our lives.

The poet and philosopher Kahlil Gibran says, "Love, like death, changes everything," and indeed it has. Our entire lives have been changed by the loss of Jamie—daughter, friend, sister, mother. The statistics regarding families that completely disintegrate following a suicide are startling. We have experienced it—the guilt, the fear, the blame, and the overwhelming feelings of helplessness. For a long time it feels as if a vital part of each of us has been amputated. There were times when I thought our family would wind up on the garbage pile of destroyed families. Now, 15 months later, I credit our decision to give the gift of life to others as being the most vital investment our family made toward our own survival, healing, and wholeness.

Death is so absolute—so final. Loving friends will offer the only comfort they can by saying, "She is not gone, she is just away." I know and appreciate all that, but the kicking, screaming child in me knows I will never brush her hair again, and we can't trade another recipe or magazine article. I can never hold her close to me again. Dead is dead! As much as you want to believe you're just having a bad dream, eventually you're left to face the reality that no matter what you do, the daughter you loved so deeply is not ever coming back.

A few weeks after Jamie's death, while I was still lost in the abyss of a bottomless emotional black hole, a letter arrived. It was from Janet Reavis of the New Mexico Donor Program. For the first time, my tears were tears of joy and comfort as I read of the lives that were enhanced—and in fact saved—because our family made Jamie's choice for her. I now know that a 48-year-old woman in San Francisco suffering from non-alcohol-related cirrhosis received Jamie's liver, and her response was very dramatic. She is married with two children. Jamie's kidneys went to two different recipients in New Mexico, each married with families. One man had waited 13 months and had become very discouraged. Janet's letter said, "Now he is a happy man."

Jamie's heart valves were used in valve replacement procedures here in New Mexico, and her pancreas was sent to the University of Miami where research in cell transplant is proving to have dramatic results in diabetes patients. Other tissue and bone were used as well, and I know that it can mean the difference between a child leaving a wheelchair or staying in it. In addition, the careers of two New Mexico men were saved by the transplant of Jamie's corneas.

Because of my deep love and commitment to children, anyone who knows me believed I was the least equipped to deal with the death of a child. Indeed, I was. I can't stress enough the part you, Dr. Lorber, and the New Mexico Donor Program have played in my own process of healing. I shudder to think where I'd be were it not for the legacy of life you and the donor program helped us to share.

Three months after Jamie died, the donor program invited me to do a television program dealing with the issue of donation. Since that program, I have assisted in making a training film for physicians and have participated in many seminars and conferences in the medical community to speak about my experience and what it has meant to me. I am an enthusiastic advocate of organ donation now and will speak wherever I am invited. We must all work together to inform and educate people not only on the wonderful medical miracles that are effected through donation, but of the comfort it brings to families to know that part of their loved one lives on. There is no greater gift. So, Dr. Lorber, my deepest thanks to you. It is my fondest hope that we all continue to work in our respective ways to further this necessary pursuit. It comes back to us in so many ways.

Please forgive the verbosity of this letter The magnitude of my feelings cannot be expressed in just a few words.

In closing I want to add—I may have lost my beloved child, but the gift of life was the only and the ultimate opportunity for a part of Jamie to live on. I was proud of her in life, and I am proud of her in death.

In gratitude,

Juliette M. Exupery
Albuquerque, New Mexico

Guidepost: The Most Difficult Crossroad

The contrast between Juliette's experience and that of the families of Bob Dale and Rick Kangas lies in the sensitivity of one caring doctor. Because of Dr. Lorber's compassion in a time of crisis for Jamie's loved ones, her gift of life lives on in many grateful recipients. And that is a deep consolation for her mother.

Sadly, the other two families were not afforded the same kindness and respect. The sister of a young donor seemed to understand why.

"When my brother died and we donated his organs, his death was the beginning of another medical procedure, and not an end in itself. I understood that so well when my grandmother died. Her organs weren't able to be donated and her death was an end. The hospital staff was wonderful in comforting and supporting us because they didn't have to deal with organ donations.

"Still, when my brother died, we needed the same kind of comfort and support, perhaps even more, but it wasn't there for us. We were pretty much told to go home and start making funeral arrangements," she said.

I had some idea of the donor process from interviewing a former organ coordinator who had given me insight into the physical pressures and psychological price of the job. "I remember the first time I did this. I walked in and thought, 'What do I say to these people? I'm sorry? I was sorry for their loss, but it was my job to ask for the organs. There were mothers of little kids who wrapped themselves around me, saying, 'Oh my god, tell me this isn't really happening!' My constant fear was that I'd walk into an intensive care unit one day and see someone I knew. I'd put my hand on the door and wonder if I could do this one more time. There were so many awful tragedies," she said.

One of the saddest, she recalled, was the young man who had been in and out of trouble and who was shot one night by the police. "When I asked his parents about donating his organs, his father said, 'Yes, it will be the only good thing he ever did.'"

She emphasized the atmosphere of urgency that surrounds the process: recipients must be found; organ donor teams are sent out to procure the organs; the organs are carefully removed and stored in ice and then are rushed to hospitals where recipients are already being prepared to receive them.

"The heart team just flies. Before leaving the operating room, I'd call the recipient hospital and give them an estimated time of arrival. But there was always the possibility of a car or plane crash, or an unexpected traffic jam that could mean a life-threatening delay," she explained.

There's also a high rate of "burn-out" in such a stress-filled job. "I finally left and vowed I'd never do it again," she said.

I recounted that interview to the young donor's sister. "Yes, that's exactly what I mean," she said. "The death of a donor is the beginning of another medical procedure and we [the donor families] get lost in it."

She was also concerned about the way in which important information was given to the donor family, stressing that medical personnel should use lay people's language when talking to the shocked and grieving family. "We need to know what brain death is and exactly how it is determined. And, we need a doctor to explain it and not pass it off to the nurses to handle. We need help to fully understand that brain death is death. I've spent years wondering if my brother was really dead," she said.

Donor families face tremendous emotional issues: Seeing a dead child or spouse who still appears to have life in the body; thinking that a loved one will become a source of organs for several donor teams with no connection or caring beyond the precision removal of body parts; and for some families, dealing with the conflict of whether or not a donation should be made.

These issues of donation remain with a donor family for a lifetime. For some, there is the haunting question, "Was it the right thing to do with our family member's body?" Others ask themselves, "Would I do this again if another tragedy occurred? Would I want my family to go through this if I died? Why can't I find consolation in giving the gift of life?"

"I don't know another donor family, but I wish I did," one spouse told me. "We're very isolated, mainly, I suppose, because there aren't many of us. I think it would be helpful if we could talk to others who have been through this."

Donor families need support groups where they can share their anguish and their consolation. Medical personnel must search for ways that they can better support the families who are willing, in the face of sudden death, to offer life.

The no-holds-barred truth is that donors are scarce. Families who feel they are treated with respect and genuine caring are likely to encourage other people to make the same generous gift. And those who feel they were treated insensitively may discourage donation. And for every donation not made, someone waiting for a transplant is closer to death.

16

Arthur: Ethics in the New Frontier

When I began research on this book, I met with many organ recipients, medical personnel, and support staff. Virtually none of them were members of an ethnic minority and I wondered why. I felt my book needed to reflect the attitudes, the fears, and hopes and dreams of people of diverse races struggling to live against difficult odds.

I began to ask questions and I've found some answers. One of the answers came through an article headlined "Study says blacks wait longer for transplants." A report by the inspector general of the Department of Health and Human Services indicated that the wait for a transplant of any organ is generally twice as long for black people as for white people, in spite of the fact that blacks are more subject to kidney failure than are whites. The article indicated that while blacks make up 12 percent of the national population, 34 percent of dialysis patients whose kidneys have failed are black. The report suggests that racial prejudice may be a factor in the longer wait.

Dr. Arthur Caplan, nationally recognized bio-medical ethicist at the University of Minnesota, concurred when I met him in his university office one afternoon.

"I do not believe that transplant centers discriminate against blacks," Dr. Caplan said. "But I think there are some quiet, subtle factors that influence the chances of blacks versus whites, that penalize blacks. One of the things that a transplant center needs to look at is the ability to pay, and since blacks have more likelihood of not having insurance because they tend to be poorer, they get excluded more from transplants.

"I think blacks are also excluded more because transplant teams take into account other questions, such as what other sicknesses, illnesses, do you have? Blacks tend to be sicker than whites because, again, they tend to be poorer and may have more diabetes, more lupis, and other diseases. So those things are against them as priorities for transplant. If we give priority to people who have closer tissue match, for kidney transplants particularly, then blacks are at a disadvantage because there aren't as many black donors, and the odds of finding a match are low.

"I suspect that if you could increase the number of minority donors, you'd go a long way toward bringing a balance. On the other hand, the only way to do that is to make sure they don't feel that the system is jerking them around. A lot of black people say, 'White people have no interest in me until I'm dead and then they want my body parts.' Until you show that you're willing to pay for health care for everybody, there will be people, particularly minorities, who feel left out and won't be altruistic.

"That's why, when states like Oregon or Arizona say they want to cut Medicaid dollars from the transplant program, it has a decimating effect on donors, especially poor people, because they think, 'If I can't get a transplant, why should I donate my organs?'

"Financing access to transplants is a way to get an increase in donors, which would then make it easier to find racial matches," Caplan said. He believes a national health care program would do just that.

Another factor in the low donor ratio may be the small number of minority organ procurement coordinators working in the seventy two organ procurement organizations. According to the report, only about fourteen of the three hundred workers are black.

Race is not the only factor in who does or doesn't get a transplant. Gender, size, and economics are also factors. Caplan points out that a woman who has been pregnant carries antibodies that make a tissue match more difficult.

Because the average woman is smaller than the average man, and because the average donor is what Caplan calls a "motorcycle male," men are more likely to get the organs. Women, he said, may often be in competition with children for organs from a small donor. And because most women work at lower paying jobs than men, they are less likely to have a health insurance plan that will cover the high costs of transplantation and aftercare.

If you're lucky enough to have a rare disease, as my sister Ardelle did, you're more likely to be of interest to a transplant center. Caplan indicated that, for research purposes, hospitals may be willing to pick up a good share of the costs of transplantation. At the time of Ardelle's surgery, she was, nationally, the second person with amyloidosis to receive a new heart.

But transplant waiting lists are growing every day. Many thousands wait for the chance to live and many die while waiting. There just aren't enough donor organs to go around, and researchers are looking at other donors besides humans. For instance, research is being done with animal hearts, including both primate and pig organs, to substitute for human hearts. But there are ethical and practical issues involved in such experimentation, Caplan believes.

"I believe there is absolutely a moral difference between using primates versus pigs. The higher up the phylogenetic scale you go, the more worth the animals have. I don't believe that fleas are worth as much as dogs or dogs worth as much as gorillas. I think it also makes a difference if an animal is becoming extinct or is abundant. Pigs are abundant and some primates, such as chimps, are not," Caplan said.

Caplan predicts very little controversy would result from the use of pig hearts because thousands are killed each year for food, but he believes using primate hearts would cause an extraordinary controversy. He also believes animals will never be used as a common source of new organs, although he thinks the animal option will be pursued in experiments. Humans, he's sure, will continue to be the optimum source.

"The psychological aspect of using animal organs can't be overlooked," he stressed.

"There are certainly issues about how we'd feel if we've got a pig heart or a cow spleen," Caplan said. "But to be blunt, I think people would accept one if it was their only way to live. They would no doubt need counseling and discussion of the issue. From talking to people who are waiting for a heart, I'm convinced that if you told them you had a good pig heart for them, they'd take it."

The other issue involved is the cost of such procedures. "While we complain because there aren't enough human organs now to transplant, the more there are, the higher the total cost. If we tripled that through the use of animal hearts, we're talking about a huge bill, and who's going to pay it?" Caplan said.

"I believe society has to pay the bill through insurance and third- party payers," he continued. "I'm convinced that we haven't vigorously pursued organ donations in this country because third party payers don't want to pick up the tab.

"The cost of these procedures should be weighed against how successful they are. In other words, what do we get for our money?

"Many other questions would have to be addressed. For instance, should children be done first; should we pick people with diseases for which there are absolutely no other options; should we take the sickest or the healthiest?"

Caplan indicated that there are about 200 centers doing heart transplants. "That's too many," he said. "The more transplants one center does, the better it gets and the better its success rate. There were about 1,400 hearts available in 1989. Some centers are probably doing only ten transplants a year, and that means they aren't doing enough to stay good at it. More people will probably die because of it. Usually, the better you are, the more cost effective you are as well.

"In Louisville, Kentucky, there are two heart transplant centers; in Philadelphia about five; in Minneapolis there are two. We probably don't need that many. It's not clear to me that there's adequate regulation and supervision of who does transplants. There may be a need for more government control. As it is, now you can just say, 'I want to be a transplant center' and you're a transplant center.

"Information should be made available to people who need a transplant, indicating which centers and even which surgeons have the best outcome ratio. I think informed consent must include that data. In most areas of medicine the consumer must rely on word of mouth or reputation," he explained.

Another practice Caplan is concerned about is called multiple listing.

"Right now, it's possible to sign up on more than one transplant center list, and that's not fair. You should only be allowed to go to one center and get on the national waiting list so you have the same chance as everyone else. In theory, there's only one list, but since organs tend to stay in the area in which they're found, it's to a person's advantage to be on the list at several centers. And the patient may not even tell one center that they're on the list at another," he said.

17

Ardelle: The Journey Comes Full Circle

After I returned from my trip with Ardelle, I called Dr. Herzog at the county medical center, explaining that doctors at Stanford had found amyloid was attacking Ardelle's new heart.

"Can I come down and talk to you?" I asked. "I want you to help me understand this disease better."

"Sure," he said. "How about Tuesday? My office, two o'clock."

"I'll be there."

I always managed to get lost while looking for his office and I was true to form. After winding through corridors and opening wrong doors, I found him.

"Hi, come on in," he said, motioning me to a chair. After showing him photos of Ardelle and Dr. Olivari, I took out my tape recorder and set it on his desk.

"I know there are different kinds of amyloid but I don't understand them very well. Explain them in simple terms," I said.

"Yes, there are several forms of amyloidosis. Ardelle has what's called 'primary amyloidosis.' It's a type of cancer of the bone marrow, producing abnormal levels of amyloid protein that's deposited in target organs.

"Then there's the familial kind that's extremely rare. That's familial Portuguese amyloid cardiomyopathy. There are about 25 families world-wide that have that disease," he said.

"What causes it?" I asked.

"We're not certain. The protein is made in the bone marrow cells, but we don't know what triggers the abnormal protein growth. The material they create has the consistency of putty. That's what Ardelle's heart was like. And when an amyloid-affected heart becomes cold, it turns very hard, like a stone," he said.

"Could any of the rest of us in the family have the primary type?"

"That's very unlikely. In the familial type, we might worry about that but not in the primary."

"It just seems so weird that she would get this disease out of nowhere."

"But that's the way it is," he said. "It's sporadic."

"What are the usual symptoms?"

"That depends on which organ is affected," he said. "Initially, with heart involvement, there is an accumulation of fluids because the mechanical properties of the ventricles are abnormal. They act as if they're very stiff.

"In the end stage, the pumping function of the heart is abnormal. That's what Ardelle had when you brought her into the hospital. She had severe, severe heart failure. And she had digitalis toxicity because she was taking digitalis for her heart condition. The amyloid actually binds the drugs and accumulates in the heart. If you hadn't brought her in, she would have died within a few days. She was in heart block for five days after she was admitted.

"She was lucky she was in Minnesota where medical assistance covers heart transplants, although I knew it would take heaven and earth to get it done in time. She was lucky, too, that Dr. Ring and Dr. Olivari were adventurous enough to do it. Many transplant centers would have said it couldn't be done.

"There certainly was academic interest in her case. But some doctors believe she shouldn't have been considered because of her age and the possibility of amyloid recurrence. But Ring made the final decision to go ahead.

"I think you knew there was some problem getting the donor heart to the hospital. It came from Ohio and had been out of the donor for four hours and eight minutes. The maximum time allowed for a heart is four hours, at least it was in 1986. Those eight minutes could have made a vital difference, but in Ardelle's case, they didn't. You know, Ring and Olivari really went out on a limb for her."

"I know they did and so did you and other people. Ardelle and the rest of us feel a great obligation to you, and we also know that this is the place where she'll get the best and the most personal care," I told him.

"Well, it all started here so we have a vested interest. And I'm going to call my debt back now. I want another echogram from her, and you can tell her she owes me one," he said, flashing a smile.

"She knows that. She's planning to come back in the spring and she'll get in touch with you when she does."

"Good," he responded.

He walked me down the hall to the elevator, and I said good-bye with a lump in my throat. This guy had set in motion the saving of Ardelle's life. Somewhere in the future we'll no doubt lose track of him, but he will remain part of our family's history by doing what he simply believed to be his job. We felt, however, he had gone quite a bit beyond.

The twins and I worried through the winter months, calling Ardelle often and listening for the tell-tale sounds of breathlessness in her voice. She was living with her daughter Julie, Julie's husband, Solie, and their three young children. We were concerned that all the activity of this lively household might exhaust her. But she seemed to weather it well.

Julie and Solie were planning to move to Minnesota, too, and would make their home in Lengby, the small town where we grew up. They had rented the tall old house just down the street from our childhood home, where the twins and I had taken piano lessons.

At the end of April, Ardelle began her trip home with a two-week stopover in Phoenix to visit Marion. Marion was shocked when she picked her up at the airport. Again she was in a wheelchair, her feet and legs swollen so badly that she couldn't wear shoes.

Two days after her arrival, Marion called to tell us that she thought Ardelle should come to Minneapolis immediately for medical care. Ardelle wouldn't hear of it. She was on her own timetable set by her knowledge of her body's clock. I think she knew there was no good reason to rush. She had planned to stay in Phoenix for two weeks, and she did, wearing expandable sandals to accommodate her swollen feet.

Then, in the second week of May, she arrived at the Twin Cities airport. It all seemed like a repeat performance for

Marilyn, Peter, and me. "Haven't we been through this before?" I quipped, as we waited for her arrival.

We found her weak and swollen but laughing and happy to see us. This time she stayed with me, my daughter Clair and our two affectionate cats, Boy and Girl. That meant walking up seven steps to the main living quarters and that was a struggle for her every time.

The day after her arrival, I stayed home from work and we made our promised pilgrimage to the medical center to give Dr. Herzog the echogram he wanted. We caught him in the midst of a busy schedule, but he quickly set up the procedure. Then he extracted a promise from us that Ardelle would go immediately to the university.

"The doctors want to see you as soon as possible," he said. "In fact, I'll call them right now and set something up."

In a half hour, the echogram was done, and we were on our way back home. "That guy doesn't fool around," I laughed.

Twice a week, I drove Ardelle to the university hospital, dropping her off at the door. Then, when her appointment ended, Marilyn would take off from work to pick her up. The doctors had given Ardelle medication to reduce the swelling, had done a heart biopsy, and had taken blood samples. Her heart, they explained, wasn't able to accept a normal blood flow because the amyloid was stiffening its walls. That's why she was retaining fluids and feeling tired. "Just getting rid of some of the swelling will make life more comfortable," they told her.

I had forewarned her that on May 17 I was having a party in honor of Senator Phil Riveness, who loved to celebrate his heritage on Norway's independence day, Syttende Mai.

"There'll be lots of people here, maybe 100 or so, and most of them will bring Scandinavian food like lefse, herring, open-faced sandwiches, and krumkake. I've got lots of work to do to get the house and the yard ready. Just hope for good weather so we can be outside for part of the evening," I told her.

On the weekend we bought boxes of flowers to plant on the patio and steps. She wanted to help me, but she didn't have the strength to do it. "You just sit and watch," I said. "There's no point in both of us getting our fingernails dirty."

I could sense the frustration she felt—this woman who had built houses and planted gardens, driven the Alcan Highway, and rescued her water-sogged photo albums from Alaskan floods.

She voiced her frustration only occasionally. But there was a poignancy in her words when she did. "Sometimes, when I hear you running up and down those steps like it was nothing, I..." her voice drifted off, but I knew the end of the sentence and I felt suddenly and deeply sad.

Ardelle's daughter Julie kept in touch by phone to report on the progress of moving the family to the house in Lengby. With Julie's next phone call from a motel near Lengby, we were both sent into depression. "Mom," she said to Ardelle, "we made it to Lengby but things don't look good. The house is falling apart, the attic is full of bat droppings, the electricity isn't turned on, and Solie's not sure if we should stay."

"Oh no," Ardelle said. "Can't you find somebody to help you do some repairs? I think you need to get some sleep and go back in the morning. Things will look better then." Ardelle hung up with a heavy sigh.

"Give them some time," I told her. "Once the house is painted and the furniture in, they'll feel differently. And once Solie sees the kids running around that big yard, he'll want to stay."

"Oh, I hope so."

I hoped so too. This tired sister of mine needed a place to settle in, to stop her traveling from one place to another, adjusting to new climates, new beds, and new floor plans. She needed a home.

May 17 dawned wet and gloomy. We decorated the house with streamers and Norwegian flags and put three leaves in the table to hold the array of food I knew would arrive. "Is Skip Humphrey really going to be here?" Ardelle asked.

"I know he's planning on it," I said. I hoped that he would attend so that she could tell the people in Lengby that she'd met the state's attorney general.

By six o'clock the rain had stopped but the grass was much too wet for outdoor entertainment. Ardelle and I slipped into our bedrooms to get dressed for the party and she came out, beaming.

"Look! I've got my black shoes on! The swelling has really gone down!" she said.

The doorbell rang as we stood admiring this pair of ordinary but wonderful black shoes. People entered, laden with bowls and platters and pans filled with delicious Scandinavian fare. And just as he had promised, Skip arrived too. He made his way around the crowded rooms, shaking hands and greeting guests. I caught him between handshakes and asked him to come in the kitchen to meet Ardelle. "She's been waiting to see you," I said.

"Hello, Ardelle," he beamed. "Happy Syttende Mai!" The two were soon discussing Norwegian ancestors, and Norwegian food and I could hear them laughing together as I piled more sandwiches unto platters. I silently blessed him for being there.

Senator Riveness arrived in time to greet most of the guests and get his musical ensemble swinging. The sounds of guitars and a base violin filled the house as people crowded around to join in singing songs both in English and Norwegian.

Ardelle was growing weary, but she hated to say good night. Finally, though, she went to bed. By one in the morning the guests were gone and the house was quiet. I sat alone for a while, unwinding from the night. This, I thought, is another of those milestones that I seem to be counting now. Next year on May 17 life would be different, I knew.

In the morning, while we had our coffee, Julie called again. There was renewed excitement in her voice. "Mom, I guess we'll stay. The house isn't quite as bad as we thought, and we can do most of the repairs ourselves. We bought some paint and Solie is laying out garden space. Some of the neighbors are going to help him get started."

"This sounds like quite a change from two days ago," Ardelle said. "I can't wait to see it. Your antique furniture should be perfect in that old house."

The news brightened her outlook and gave her a surge of energy. "I'd like to buy some presents to take to Lengby with me. Let's go shopping," she said.

"Okay. What if we stop at a few garage sales? We might find some old things that would just fit in the house," I said.

Each stop was a struggle for her: getting in the car, getting out of the car, walking up the drive-ways, scouring the tables of left-over treasures. But we found just the things we were looking for.

There was a little red lantern and a Dresden blue pitcher that would be perfect for daisies. And there were straw holders for paper plates. "We can use them for our family reunion," she said.

Ardelle had announced earlier that she was planning a family reunion to be held on July 6 in Lengby. "I want everybody to come. Jon and his family will be here from Seattle, and brother Bud promised he'd come, too. I told the doctors to keep me alive until then, but they said I'd keep myself alive. I'll really be disgusted if I don't make it!"

"Oh, you'll make it," I assured her.

She sent out invitations to relatives we hadn't seen for years and began planning the menu. "We'll have it at Julie's. She's got a big yard, and we'll borrow some picnic tables. Everybody can bring something to eat, just like at your party, and if they want to stay overnight, they can sleep on the floor in sleeping bags."

On May 19, we packed her suitcases, hiding our garage sale treasures inside, and began the next leg of her journey back home. We were to meet our brother Darrell and his wife Liz about an hour out of Minneapolis for breakfast. They would take Ardelle to their home. Then, the following Tuesday, a cousin would deliver her to Lengby. That way, the trip would be broken up and it would give her time to visit relatives.

Marilyn and I kissed Ardelle good-bye in the restaurant parking lot and watched our brother drive away, with Ardelle waving from the back seat.

I put my arm around Marilyn. "It's been a long journey, but she's almost home," I said.

Epilogue
Saying Farewell

On August 21, 1991, as the world watched the Soviet Union struggle for its freedom, Ardelle slipped quietly into her own freedom. Her daughter Julie was by her side.

Once more my family made its way to Lengby. It was there Ardelle had chosen to return when death could no longer be deferred by miracles.

When we arrived at Julie and Solie's home, friends and neighbors were already there, offering sympathy and food in immeasurable quantities, and engulfing us in love.

Ardelle's last wishes were that her heart be removed for medical research and that she be cremated and buried near our parents and infant sister. She wanted a simple service that remembered our life with her. We honored all those wishes.

On the evening before the memorial, my daughter, Clair, and two of her cousins gathered flowers from a neighbor's garden—gladiolas in pink, white, orange, and yellow, and crysanthemums in rusty orange and pink. And in the morning we carried them to a little chapel and placed them near a photo album that held remembrances of Ardelle's life.

In a eulogy, Marilyn recalled our most precious childhood moments with Ardelle, beginning with that special memory of cuddling together on the bed, listening to her reading stories and poems in the dim light of evening.

Then we read a poem for her. We had chosen one that I had written when our mother died. I remembered

Ardelle saying, "I like that poem. It's the way I think about death." I offer it here, in memory of our courageous Ardelle:

> *When you are told that death has come for me,*
> *Do not believe it.*
> *Walk among the trees and I will speak to you*
> *In the soft, mystery song of the wind.*
> *Touch a leaf sprinkled with sunshine*
> *And you will be touching me.*
> *Pick up a smooth, worn stone and throw it far*
> *Into the sea.*
> *That will help you to understand that I am not dead:*
> *Whether I am in your hand*
> *Or in the sea,*
> *I am a Child of the Changing Earth,*
> *Changed and free.*

Chronimed Publishing Books of Related Interest

☐ **When You're Sick and Don't Know Why: Coping with Your Undiagnosed Illness** by Linda Hanner, John J. Witek, M.D., with Robert B. Clift, Ph.D. This warm and comprehensive guide offers hope and practical advice for dealing with an undiagnosed illness and for obtaining an accurate diagnosis as quickly as possible.
"Reassuring, helpful, and broadly applicable." —Mary Hager, Newsweek
004087, ISBN 0-937721-83-2, $9.95

☐ **Diagnosing Your Doctor** by Arthur R. Pell, Ph.D. Authoritative, straightforward, and powerful, this book tells how to get the most from doctors and medical professionals—and shows you how to ask tough questions to get the right answers.
004090, ISBN 0-937721-87-5, $9.95

☐ **Minute Health Tips: Medical Advice and Facts at a Glance** by Thomas Welch, M.D. This valuable and easy-to-use guide discusses routine health problems, offers preventive medicine tips, shows you how to make doctor visits more informational, and much more.
004088, ISBN 0-937721-85-9, $8.95

☐ **Doctor, Why Do I Hurt So Much?** by Mark H. Greenberg, M.D., Lucille Frank, M.D., & Jackson Braider. This revolutionary guide will show you how to find relief from symptoms of over 100 different types of arthritis (and dozens of other related illnesses) as well as the causes.
004091, ISBN 0-937721-88-3, $14.95

☐ **Emergency Medical Treatment: Infants— A Handbook of What to Do in an Emergency to Keep an Infant Alive Until Help Arrives** by Stephen Vogel, M.D., and David Manhoff, produced in cooperation with the National Safety Council. This easy-to-follow, step-by-step guide tells exactly what to do during the most common, life-threatening situations you might encounter for infants. Fully illustrated and indexed with thumb tabs.
004582, ISBN 0-916363-01-5, $7.95

☐ **Emergency Medical Treatment: Children— A Handbook of What to Do in an Emergency to Keep a Child Alive Until Help Arrives** by Stephen Vogel, M.D., and David Manhoff, produced in cooperation with the National Safety Council. This easy-to-follow, step-by-step guide tells exactly what to do during the most common, life-threatening situations you might encounter for children. Fully illustrated and indexed with thumb tabs.
004583, ISBN 0-916363-00-7, $7.95

☐ **Emergency Medical Treatment: Adults— A Handbook of What to Do in an Emergency to Keep an Adult Alive Until Help Arrives** by Stephen Vogel, M.D., and David Manhoff, produced in cooperation with the National Safety Council. This easy-to-follow, step-by-step guide tells exactly what to do during the most common, life-threatening situations you might encounter for adults. Fully illustrated and indexed with thumb tabs.
004584, ISBN 0-916363-05-8, $7.95

☐ **The Physician Within** by Catherine Feste. Here internationally renowned health motivation specialist, Cathy Feste, focuses on motivating those with a health challenge, and anyone else, to stay on their regimen and follow healthy behavior.
004019, ISBN 0-937721-19-0, $8.95

☐ **Whole Parent/Whole Child: A Parent's Guide to Raising a Child with a Chronic Illness** by Patricia Moynihan, R.N., P.N.P., M.P.H., and Broatch Haig, R.D., C.D.E. Everything parents of children with chronic health conditions need to know is here. With authority, insight, and compassion, this book shows you how to be the kind of parent you want to be and how to help your child lead the fullest life possible.
004051, ISBN 0-937721-53-0, $9.95

☐ **I Can Cope: Staying Healthy with Cancer** by Judi Johnson, R.N., Ph.D., and Linda Klein. This book is a clear, comprehensive resource for anyone whose life has been touched by cancer. And it's by Judi Johnson, co-founder of the American Cancer Society's internationally acclaimed "I Can Cope" program, which helps over 40,000 people a year.
004026, ISBN 0-937721-28-X, $8.95

☐ **Making the Most of Medicare: A Personal Guide Through the Medicare Maze** by Arthur R. Pell, Ph.D. Finally, a book that actually helps overcome the government red tape associated with Medicare. It shows what can and cannot be expected from Medicare and provides easily understood explanations of Medicare policies—plus tips on how to use them for optimum advantage.
004071, ISBN 0-937721-66-2, $11.95

☐ **Retirement: New Beginnings, New Challenges, New Successes** by Leo Hauser and Vincent Miller. From two internationally renowned motivational speakers, trainers, and retirees comes a book that will help you achieve new goals in retirement. It's a plan of action that charts a course to successful, rewarding, and active retirement.
004059, ISBN 0-937721-59-X, $5.95

☐ **Fast Food Facts** by Marion Franz, RD. This revised and up-to-date bestseller shows how to make smart nutritional choices at fast food restaurants—and tells what to avoid. Includes complete nutrition information on more than 1,000 menu offerings from the 32 largest fast food chains.
Standard-size edition   004068, ISBN 0-937721-67-0, $6.95
Pocket edition   004073, ISBN 0-937721-69-7, $4.95

☐ **Convenience Food Facts** by Arlene Monk, RD. Includes complete nutrition information, tips, and exchange values on over 1,500 popular name-brand processed foods commonly found in grocery store freezers and shelves. It helps you plan easy-to-prepare, nutritious meals.
004081, ISBN 0-937721-77-8, $10.95

☐ **All-American Low-Fat Meals in Minutes** by M.J. Smith, RD, LD, MA. Filled with tantalizing recipes and valuable tips, this cookbook makes great-tasting low-fat foods a snap for holidays, special occasions, or everyday. Most recipes take only minutes to prepare.
004079, ISBN 0-937721-73-5, $12.95

☐ **All-American Low-Fat Meals in Minutes** by M.J. Smith, RD, LD, MA. Filled with tantalizing recipes and valuable tips, this cookbook makes great-tasting low-fat foods a snap for holidays, special occasions, or everyday. Most recipes take only minutes to prepare.
004079, ISBN 0-937721-73-5, $12.95

☐ **Healing the Body Betrayed** by Robert A. Klein, Ph.D., and Marcia Goodman Landau, Ph.D. This self-paced guide shows how to regain psychological control of your chronic illness — and how to live the fullest life possible.
004098, ISBN 1-56561-003-2, $12.95

Buy them at your local bookstore or use this convenient coupon for ordering.

CHRONIMED Publishing
P.O. Box 47945
Minneapolis, MN 55447-9727

Please send me the books I have checked above. I am enclosing $_____. (Please add $2.50 to this order to cover postage and handling. Minnesota residents add 6.5% sales tax.) Send check or money order, no cash or C.O.D.'s. Prices are subject to change without notice.

Name _____

Address _____

City _____ State _____ Zip _____

Allow 4 to 6 weeks for delivery.
Quantity discounts available upon request.

Or order by phone: 1-800-848-2793,
1-800-444-5951 (non-metro area of Minnesota)
612-541-0239 (Minneapolis/St. Paul metro area).

Please have your credit card number ready.